Aging, Health Care, And You!

A Doctor's Personal Prescription for Understanding and Improving Your Health Care

Lessons, Insights, and Informative Practical Guidance for the Aging Health Care Consumer

BY MARTIN S. FINKELSTEIN, MD, FACP

ISBN: 1470061945

ISBN 13: 9781470061944

Library of Congress Control Number: 2012903109

CreateSpace, North Charleston, SC

A Person Can Grow Old Trying to Stay Young!

As we age, the struggle to maintain health and youth keeps getting more complex, keeps requiring more effort, and eventually wears us out. You might as well resign yourself to reality and enjoy what you are and what you have.

Comments from older health care consumers and readers

"An informative and comforting book that belongs on the night table in every home for quick and easy reference"

"For me, old age began at ninety, and I had no idea how to handle it—I wish I had the book at that time."

"Must reading for every senior and those coming of age"

"Read this book and add years to your life— learn to cope with all that comes your way"

"Dr. Finkelstein demystifies the aging process and then offers the practical advice that has enabled me and other grateful patients to remain active, self-reliant, and healthy enough to experience the unique joys and compensations of a long life."

"This book is an extremely valuable resource for anyone over sixty-five. It provides a complete compendium of issues that one may face in the normal process of aging."

"The author actually understands the problems of aging. He has wisdom and compassion and offers the reader specific, practical ways of coping."

"Aging, Health Care and You! is a must-read for every American over fifty years of age."

"This book is a valuable resource. It tells us what we need to know, but is not always comfortable to ask."

"[Aging, Health Care and You!] is packed with useful information, extraordinary insights, and is written in an easy-to-understand format."

Dedication

This book is dedicated to the memory of the best physician
I ever met, and the person who taught me the most of what
it means to be a caring doctor and a compassionate human
being—a mensch:
–Hyman M. Finkelstein, MD—my father.

And to the memory of my late close colleague and friend,
Dr. Michael L. Freedman, with whom I shared an office and a
career, and who for thirty-five years directed Geriatrics at NYU
Medical Center, was a leader in geriatric medical training and
education, and taught me much of what aging was all about.
This book represents a synthesis of many of the topics and
discussions we pondered and shared over the past decades.

Acknowledgements

I would like to thank and express my appreciation to my wife, Diana, for her tolerance, assistance, and encouragement while I was working on this manuscript.

I am forever grateful for the training and teaching of my professors and mentors: Dr. Jonathan Uhr, Dr. Thomas Merigan, Dr. Saul J. Farber, and Dr. H. Sherwood Lawrence.

I thank all my patients, who, over the past forty-seven years, taught me what was really important in medicine and what really mattered to them and their families, and who honored and entrusted me with caring for their lives.

And a very special thanks to my patients Barbara Brett, who gave me early guidance and encouragement in publishing this book; and Harris Schoenberg, who reviewed the manuscript as a consumer, and who painstakingly found and corrected so many grammatical and language errors.

Illustrations and Diagrams: by Alejandro Mazon

Table of Contents

Page

INTRODUCTION

SECTION I — AGING

Fear of Aging —"I don't want to get old!"	1
Understanding Aging	4
So why do we have to age?	4
How Old is "Old"?	8
The Lasting Scars of the Past	8
How fast do we Age?	12
How important is Greater Longevity?	13
How do we Age?	14
How our body composition changes with age	18
How elderly are viewed— common stereotypes	19
What should be our Goals of Living?	21
Making Priorities and Life Choices	23

SECTION II — ILLNESS AND HEALTH

Medical Aspects Associated with Aging	37
What You Should Know about Illness and Hospitalization	38
Managing an Unexpected Sudden Illness	41

Risks of Surgery in the Elderly 42

The Impact and Challenge of Stroke 45

Feeling of Weakness and Generalized Fatigue 49

Feeling Unsteady: Balance, Falling and Hip Fractures 51

Feeling Dizzy and Having Black Outs 55

Suffering with Insomnia and Sleep Disturbances 59

Feeling Numbness and Tingling in the Fingers 63

Annoying Tremors and Shaking in Your Hands 66

Having a Degenerative Disease 67

Fear of Dementia 68

The Cloud of Depression 75

Significance of Heart Failure and Palpitations 77

The Predictive Value of Screening for Cardiovascular
    Disease 81

Detecting Swollen Legs and Feet 84

Pain in the Legs while Walking, and Circulation Problems 89

The Agony of Leg Cramps 92

Getting Short of Breath with Doing Nothing 94

Bothered by a Chronic and Recurrent Cough 96

The "Shadow" of Cancer 99

Suffering with Back Pain and Sciatica 104

Aching with Arthritis; Painful Hips, Knees,
    and Shoulders 110

Suffering with Painful Feet 114

Afraid of "Collapsing" with Osteoporosis 116

The Curse of Constipation 123

Experiencing Gas and Abdominal Distention 126

Experiencing Heartburn, Reflux and Chest Pain 129

Trouble Swallowing and Aspirating Food and Liquid 133

Another Bladder Infection and Other Urinary Problems 135

Aspects of Infections and Fever in the Elderly 138

Seeing "ugly" Lesions on Your Skin, and Hair Thinning 144
Why do we Get Pressure Ulcers? 147
Those Annoying Drying Conditions 150
Unhappy with Your Weight 152
Hardships of Living Disabled 154
Important Family Concerns 157
The Goal of Healthy Living 161

SECTION III — BEING AN OLDER PATIENT

Reducing Confusion Taking Medications 172
Making Sense of Test Results 182
Trying to Figure Out Your Health Insurance Coverage 187
Understanding Coding and Medical Billing 196
Surviving Hospitalization 200
Struggling with End of Life Decisions 209
Need for Care 209
Understanding and Making Advance Directives 212
Teaming and Interacting with Your Doctor 215
Hiring a Doctor 215
Cooperative Interacting with Your Doctor 217
Being an Informed Patient and Smarter Consumer 223
Managing Medical Emergencies 225
Current and Future Issues in Health Care 227
Advocacy and Allegiance 227
Finances Control the Health Care System 229
The Challenge of Defending our Humanity 232
New Directions in Therapy 236
Drowning in Information Overload 241

SECTION IV — SUMMARY AND CONCLUSIONS 245

INDEX 251

Glossary of Medical Words 257

About the Author 261

Introduction

Old age though despised, is coveted by all.

PROVERB

"Pills and bills - Leaks and squeaks!" Is this what getting older is all about? Older people have a wide assortment of very troubling issues that keep recurring; issues regarding their healthcare and their actual physical and mental health.

With the aches and pains that seem to affect every part of the body, and with all the medical issues, fears, and concerns that escalate with aging, older patients require much medical attention and caring. However, with today's health care, patients may have only 10-15 minutes of face-time with their doctor during any outpatient office or clinic visit (and face time is likely to decrease in the future). This is far too little time to address the multiple complex medical problems that confound the elderly. It is not nearly enough time to answer and deal with their most important questions and issues. This book was written to fill many of the gaps in their knowledge, and help our seniors (and those caring for them) to understand what's happening in their bodies and in their medical life. This book confronts the complexity of health care for the elderly: explaining illness and health, treatment and medical care, hospitals and medical insurance.

"Old age ain't no place for sissies"—a quote from Bette Davis may fundamentally be true, but the stress and medical consequences of aging can be made more manageable by being better informed. Knowledge is empowerment! Everyone ages, and we usually hate being reminded of this basic fact of life. Never have we been as old as we are at present, and having had no personal experience of what being this old entails, each new day brings some uncertainty regarding our body's health. Every new ache can therefore be met with anxiety about what it portends. We see problems of older relatives and friends and worry about what will happen to us when we get to be their age. When a contemporary dies, we suddenly feel older and more vulnerable. Who will take care of us if we, or our spouse, become feeble and unable to function independently? Facing the problems expected with advanced age is often an abstract exercise for younger people, but is a very tangible reality for the older generation. Many emotions run through our minds when we think about getting old ourselves. Understanding what's happening is key to being prepared and in control.

Over the past several decades, health care has changed in fundamental and dramatic ways. It is now big business. Gone are the days of the neighborhood GP (or general practitioner, the local private doctor, who knew you and your family intimately, made house calls, and who performed all needed medical care from the delivery of babies to small surgeries in his office). Gone are the days of the small independent doctor-run hospital that was located near your home, and where you were made to feel at home. No matter how much they might prefer, doctors no longer can schedule enough face time with patients to address all their troubling questions and issues during a single visit.

Older attitudes and older ways of delivering health care are obsolete. The complexity of today's medical care has spawned syndicates and industries that did not previously exist. The complexity of care extends to areas of testing, procedures, innovative treatments; models of medical care delivery, medical insurance, and the places where health care is delivered. Indeed, every aspect of medical care has changed and has become far more complex since the time older people were young. Health care today is an enormous, complex industry, with many components, many competing agendas, and with vast economic and political ramifications.

Although the elderly are the major consumers of medical care, they are among the least prepared for dealing with the reality of today's health care system. They remain more attuned to how medicine was practiced decades ago. Many seniors feel that medical care today is missing the personal relationship they once had with the doctor who knew them as a person, not just a disease. As a result, older people are often overwhelmed by medical and social challenges that confront them when they become ill. They often have difficulties in getting assistance when trying to deal with their health, and most need some assistance and guidance to navigate their way. This responsibility often falls to family and friends, who may themselves be confused by the bureaucracy of our current health system.

Not only has medical care become more complex, the actual medical problems of older patients become more complex. Past illnesses and experiences leave their imprints on the body. And since every organ and structure has aged, every body component is more vulnerable to the burdens of illness. The impressive functional reserve we had with youth, and the capacity to tolerate the stress of illness and heal quickly, has been significantly deteriorated by aging. Simple diseases often disturb many different body functions. With newer technology and more sensitive tools, doctors can reveal the accumulated damage of past stressful events, but the task of relating these discoveries to the specific problems of the patient can become a major challenge. Social and financial problems associated with being ill have become more complex. Caring for the elderly is probably the most complex type of care faced in today's complex health-care system.

With an aging population, and longer life expectancy, we can expect the changes that are happening in medicine today to become more profound in the future. Financial issues are now having a powerful impact in directing the focus of health care.

What I have done in this guide to aging is to write down many of my observations and thoughts about what is important to most of us as we age. This is condensed from my more than than sixty-five years of personally observing the changes in medicine (starting as a child growing up in a house where my father conducted a general medical practice) and including thirty-seven years of practicing and teaching geriatrics at a major medical center in New York; teaching doctors, geriatricians, nurses, students, and, most importantly, my patients. It condenses what my patients have taught me over my many years in clinical practice. These are my responses and explanations to the most common complaints and problems that I have witnessed repeatedly in people as they age: problems older patients encounter regularly in the hospital and in doctor's offices; problems and issues which disturb them, and about which they repeatedly complain and seek help and guidance.

The elderly population is very heterogeneous, and my recommendations and comments may not be applicable to all seniors or families of seniors. But it is clear that a very sizeable percentage of our elderly seem unprepared for the experiences that await them when they become ill and must interact with today's medical system. They need information and greater understanding.

I believe everyone should have a basic understanding of what is going on in their bodies, and why they experience the complaints they do. It is *their* body, and they should know what's wrong with it, and what it is that's responsible for their complaints. In fact, since it is their body, they have *more* of a right to know what's going on than does anyone else. I have had need to explain basic medical issues repeatedly to patients over the years, and have realized that patients want explanations for what's happening in their bodies. But lacking an understanding of disease, and perhaps being too embarrassed to discuss their health issues with their busy doctor, many are left hungry for information, and appreciate the explanations of why they feel the way they do. I believe that being better informed about what it is that bothers them makes people better patients, and smarter consumers of health care. Indeed, any consent to treatment (implied or written) would require the patient be adequately informed about choices and options, and understand the consequences of their decision.

I have separated the material in this book into three sections: Aging in general, and problems associated by everyone as they age; specific illnesses and medical problems that have special significance to the elderly; and practical issues with the logistics of health-care delivery for older patients.

This guide represents my attitudes and perspective on various health issues encountered by the older patient, and emphasizes what people should know but may not understand about their bodies and about health care. It is what I believe are the key elements that they and their families should understand in order to minimize the problems they regularly encounter with their health care. People reading this book are welcome to share or reject my viewpoints, but at least they should think about the issues I enumerate, and make their own choices.

Our population is aging due to aging of the baby boomers and to our lengthening life expectancy. There have been many books written about various aspects of aging; and there are websites that contain complex information to explain, or extend a reader's understanding of the researched problem. Sometimes too much information can be confusing and overwhelming. In this book, it has been my older patients' observed problems that have determined the subject matter, and the explanations that seemed to help and clarify the confusion that formed the basis of my counsel.

This book is not intended to be a textbook in geriatric medicine, nor a comprehensive, authoritative reference manual, but rather a practical guide for older people and families caring for older relatives. It cannot, nor does not, cover every medical problem affecting the elderly; but rather, the scope is limited to what has bothered my patients most commonly. Its intent is to offer lessons, insights, and practical guidance for the consumer, providing greater understanding of what aging and health care is now about.

The information contained in this book should help you to understand the complexities of today's health care in the US. Some may find the information too detailed and too complex for them to fully appreciate. Others may find the information incomplete, too simple, and not meeting their expectations. I recommend people read those sections that interest them most, but also try to gain a sense of what problems their bodies will encounter as they age. Generally, people are widely divided in how well they process medical information, how interested they are in absorbing such information, or, if they have not had any scientific background, a fear of being overwhelmed by exposure to "health sciences." I have tried to tread a middle ground at a level at which, over the years, I have found most of my patients seem to grasp and appreciate the information contained in this book. It is my belief that *any* improvements in people's grasp of basic medical facts will help them become better patients, and help them with their medical care in the long run. It may also save them money.

Basic health care is far too important to entrust to others to manage without any involvement by the patients themselves. It is my purpose to make you a more informed patient, and offer guidance to a longer and happier life.

SECTION I — AGING

Seek ye counsel of the aged for their eyes have looked on the faces of the years and their ears have hardened to the voices of Life. Even if their counsel is displeasing to you, pay heed to them.

KAHLIL GIBRAN

Fear of Aging — "I Don't Want to Get Old!"

Fearing aging is another way of actually saying that you fear staying alive. However, many are afraid of aging—but why? It is the most natural thing in the world. You have only to keep living to age. "We should only live long enough." There is only one alternative to aging, and that one is usually not the acceptable choice. If we're lucky, we all will get to be old. The very fact that a person has gotten older proves that the person has a pretty good body, has survived and "made it" for many years, and may well do so for many more.

Young children today often seek out the advice and support of their grandparents or older relatives, as their advice and guidance usually comes without criticism, but rather in a supportive and comforting manner. Throughout history, the aged were respected, even venerated. They were admired for their wisdom and understanding of life, and how and why things worked. Because of their accumulated wisdom and experience, they offered a perspective that younger people lacked; and thus the aged were in demand. The elderly were usually no longer concerned with their own self-advancement, but rather sought more on how to assist and help others by sharing their accumulated knowledge and wisdom. They no longer needed to compete, nor be so concerned with what others thought of them; they had no need to prove themselves. They were not feared, nor were they scorned. They had earned their place in society. Until infirmity limited their capacity, they were the accepted leaders of the tribe or society.

Why, then, should we now fear getting old? Why are the elderly the butt of so many jokes? By joking about it, do we gain some psychological control over aging and make it less frightening? Is it that we mourn the passing of our youth, or that with age, most of our life is now behind us? Is it that our bodies can no longer do what they used to do, or that opportunities for "remaking" our lives (particularly if we are disappointed in the life we have) become less likely? We may also fear being alone and lonely at an older age—having lost our peers, friends, or partners. We all recognize that our time will come, and we may mourn the loss of some aspects of youth, but despite the aging of our bodies, we have a lot to be proud of and never should feel the need to apologize or be ashamed for being old or living a long life.

Is the concept of dying becoming more palpable and real, and what we fear with aging is the process of dying or being dead? The reasons for fearing one's own aging may differ between people, but the fear of aging as a concept, and trying to deny or fight aging, is very common in the "not so very old." It is the younger individual who often fears getting old; the older person, who experiences what "old" entails, is rarely afraid of getting older (nor of being dead)—they fear becoming ill, with all it's anticipated ramifications.

We are all familiar with mid-age crises that many people experience in their forties, fifties, or sixties, but we don't see this same anxiety in the older population. There is a peace and tranquility that should come with aging and resignation to the reality of no longer being young. Aging still brings experience and greater wisdom to many, at least till the systems start breaking down. What older people seem to fear most about getting older is the debility we see in the very old; becoming a physical, financial, and emotional burden on those they care most about; or that when very old, they will suffer with pain and indignity for a considerable period. Children and grandchildren usually fear aging in their older relative far more than does the older relative herself. The very existence and presence of a parent is comforting, and seems a shield against the child's own mortality. Children fear the parent's absence and debility at least as keenly as does the older person.

In the past, humans always lived in extended family situations. While living in the same cave, tent, or within small tribal communities, life's changes were manifest to all, and were probably better understood and accepted than they are now. Birth, death, illness, and aging were considered neither mysterious nor abnormal, but rather part of normal life processes. In developed countries today, we frequently isolate the elderly or infirm from the rest of the community, making the changes that occur with aging or infirmity something more mysterious, fearful, and unknown.

Would we like to be like Dorian Grey, who, in the story by Oscar Wilde, remains handsome and youthful while only his portrait shows his life's stress? How many of us would like never to age or mature? And how old would we like to remain? We may not like it, but we should not fear aging. At any age of life, it's best to adjust to the conditions imposed by aging, enjoy its rewards, and deal with its problems.

Understanding Aging

So why do we have to age?

Aging is one of the most natural, but least understood events in nature. All living things age! Actually, everything in the universe ages: rocks, mountains, our planet, our sun, the universe. Nothing stays the same throughout time. In living organisms, aging is the natural progression of maturing. The newborn infant, who grows and matures, is *really* in fact aging. There is no boundary line between *maturing* and *aging.* It's not even clear whether aging is a smooth continuum or occurs in a small step-wise manner throughout life.

On the surface, we recognize that some forms of life never seem to age or die. Bacteria can divide and can perpetuate seemingly identical clones of them indefinitely, given adequate food supply and space for them to grow. But mutations do occur that sometimes are fatal and become the end of the line for that particular single-celled organism. Individual bacterial cells do not live forever. Some cancers and tumor cells can similarly divide and replicate forever, given favorable growth conditions; but individual cells do not live forever. There is, however, a major difference between these cells and our own. Taken out of our bodies, our own individual cells cannot replicate and divide indefinitely, even if given nourishment and space. There are a programmed number of divisions that our "normal" cells have, after which they no longer can divide.

In our own bodies, cells have their own life expectancy, and are replaced at the end of their programmed life. Different types of cells have markedly different life expectancies. We are constantly turning over cells, so that newly formed cells continually replace senescent or outdated cells. This is critical to our existence. Some cells, such as blood-forming cells and cells lining our gastrointestinal tract have relatively short turnovers (or shortened life expectancy). As a result, these cells are the most susceptible to agents that affect cell division (such as many anticancer drugs). Other cells, such as nerve cells, grow and replace themselves very slowly. Aging is not random, and there is a natural programmed age and death that exists in all living things, from individual cells to whole organisms.

We recognize that some trees, and giant mold (or fungus) seem to live for thousands of years, but the individual cells making up the mold or tree need replacement. Still, the structure of the living mass seems to survive for long, long periods.

As science unravels the mysteries governing the cycles of growth, life, and repair, we are gaining more understanding of the processes of energy renewal, mitochondrial function, genetic replication, and programmed cell death, all of which seem essential for life and are part of the aging process.

There are different theories of what causes aging: A mitochondrial theory states that mitochondria[1] (which are the energy factories within our cells) lose their number and function as we age. Mitochondria lack the capacity to replace themselves indefinitely, as they cannot repair defects and mutations in their own genes as they occur, thus leading to their eventual loss. They are the sites of greatest oxidative stress. With the loss of these energy factories, the animal slowly loses the energy needed to

---

1 Mitochondria are living subcellular organisms in all dividing cells, and have their own genes and DNA. They are the site of ATP production, the energy needed for life.

sustain life. One of the hallmarks of aging is fatigue and generalized weakness. Another theory holds that the loss of telomeres, small attachments to our DNA, which allow replication of our genes, is responsible for aging. With succeeding replications, these telomeres are lost, until there are not enough available to allow cell replacement. Another theory holds that with aging, membranes and proteins may not be adequately removed and digested, which leads to an accumulation of inactive partially denatured material that interferes with the normal functioning of the active proteins and membranes. Aging is a consequence of continually accumulated damaged cells and materials that affect all life processes. Mutational theories hold that if our stem cells acquire enough mutations, they can no longer function or replace damaged cells. Still another mutational theory claims that small mutations and changes in our cells and proteins confuse our bodies to identify the "abnormal" or aged cells as "foreign" and something that should be removed. We do realize that mutations are not random, and that there are "hot" spots in our genes that have a much higher mutational frequency. Probably all of these aging problems occur to one degree or another. New understanding of aging will no doubt arise from current and future research about life's processes.

Still, there is the attraction of retarding the aging process; staying young, active, and virile, to the envy of our peers (as if drinking from The Fountain of Youth). We would all like to retain all the vigor and youthful appearance we had when younger. There have been a number of studies that have explored the age-retarding effects of various hormones, whose production decreases dramatically with aging. These include: human growth hormone, estrogens, androgens (the male hormones), and DHEA (an adrenal hormone that is converted mostly into estrogens and androgens). The results of these studies have been mostly disappointing, with inconsistent results, or showing an increased risk of serious medical health problems. This is why they are not being promoted for any anti-aging effect at this time. Mostly, these are the same hormones that are banned for use by competitive athletes, and for which drug testing has been endorsed. The general wisdom is that these hormones are best used under careful medical supervision in individuals with documented hormone deficiency states. There is an increased risk of acquiring various cancers with their administration (particularly with unmonitored administration). Growth hormone can also raise blood pressure, injure muscles, promote fluid retention, and affect heart muscle. Androgens are listed as restricted drugs (similar to narcotics), to reduce abuse. Androgens can lower the good cholesterol (HDL) in the blood, while raising the bad LDL. Androgens stimulate prostate growth, raise blood pressure, increase hair loss, affect heart muscle, increase the risk of tendon rupture, and encourage clotting. In younger men, it will suppress fertility. DHEA can be purchased from health food and vitamin stores, but the preparations are unregulated, and the anti-aging value, unproved. Estrogens can increase clots in leg veins, stimulate growth of the uterine lining and breast tissue (with the fear of increasing breast and uterine cancer development).

Another technique for preserving a youthful appearance is the local injection of botulinum toxin (Botox) into facial muscles. This procedure has become popular for reducing facial and neck wrinkles. The toxin weakens injected muscles, causing them to relax, thus diminishing the wrinkle. When performed by an experienced provider, the technique is relatively safe and effective, but requires a series of injections, and the benefits are only temporary (measured in months). Repeated series of injections will be needed to extend the beneficial effect. Insurance companies generally do not pay for cosmetic procedures.

How old is "old"?

There is no accepted definition of the word *old* in medicine. The term *old* or *aged* is ambiguous. Sometimes the word *senior* is considered less distasteful. The word *senile*, of course, carries bad connotations. Ask a teenager when a person is "old," and they might say, "Thirty-five." Ask a seventy-year-old the same question, and he may reply, "Eighty-five." Cultural differences also affect responses. In India, Japan, New Guinea, and different regions of the US, one might get very different responses. *Aged* and *old* are relative terms, and are perceived by the individuals responding according to the general age of the population around them. In a world of toddlers, a teenager would feel old. The expression "You are as old as you feel" might be a very accurate portrayal of how a person views his or her own age. Some people seem young at eighty-five, others old at fifty. Much of aging is attitude. If you ask older individuals if they dream, and how old they are in their dreams, one gets startling results that separate individuals according to how they view their health and age when they are awake. This seems to reflect their self-image—how they feel about themselves. We all have self-images that do not age gradually. Our self-image ages in sudden steps when an illness or accident reveals our shortcomings and inability to respond or recuperate the way we would have imagined.

The lasting scars of the past

Being older means having already lived for a considerable time in the past. The health implications of this obvious fact are frequently not well understood by many who see the world only in today's terms, or who are not familiar with history or the environments that existed decades ago. Consider what living conditions were like some fifty, sixty, or seventy years ago. Consider also where the older individual was born, and under what conditions they previously lived. They might well have received childhood therapies and exposures that we can't even imagine today. Such conditions can make vast imprints upon an older person's later medical status.

Living conditions, common infections, environmental exposures, working conditions (including lack of limitations on the length of the workweek, or union-demanded worker's rights), and dietary limitations (particularly during wars and periods of famine, when starvation was common), were far different than those that now exist in the US. Older people bear the scars of these exposures, emotionally and physically. Diseases like polio, TB, and diphtheria were common in the developed world. Wartime exposures in allied soldiers, as well as in victims of wars, frequently led to problems with typhus, typhoid, malaria, trench foot, frostbite, TB, trachoma, and vascular disease. In some regions of the world, parasitic infections were the norm. With past economic depressions and wars, deep psychic scars left an indelible mark. Intense psychic and emotional scars were also etched by the greater racial and religious intolerance that existed at the time.

Diets and presence of environmental toxins were very different than today. Fresh vegetables and fruit were available in season only, or they were frozen. Smoking, eating heavily fried foods, drinking alcohol, and smoking during pregnancy were not considered hazardous. Smoking was not banned in public spaces, and "passive" smoking in bars, offices, restaurants, and even hospitals was unavoidable. People did not concern themselves with cholesterol or a need to exercise. Mercury, lead, and asbestos were commonly used by everyone in schools, at work, and at home without fear. Silver was often used to treat sores and wounds. Food and water were not tested for contamination by toxic chemicals or for infectious agents. No environmental protection group existed to regularly monitor the air, water, and food for pollution. In dental offices, doctor's offices, and even in shoe stores (where children could stand under fluoroscopy—X-ray—machines for hours admiring their skeletal feet), people were exposed to large doses of X-rays in amounts much greater than they are today. X-ray "treatments" were common for management of acne and skin disorders. X-ray treatment was even used to treat infections and abscesses in the lung. There were no regulatory restrictions on safety conditions in the workplace or at home. Even in medicine, mercury was regularly injected into patients as the most commonly used diuretic for treating heart failure or edema. Radon was commonly placed on watches to make the numbers and watch hands glow in the dark. Reusable needles and syringes were the norm, and were often inadequately sterilized by quick exposure to boiling water before being reused on other people. This would not have been adequate to kill many pathogens, and probably as a result, hepatitis virus exposure was almost universal, as judged by the prevalence of immunity to hepatitis viruses found in older people throughout the world. Unless you were a government employee, veteran, or Native American, your health insurance (if you had any) was likely to be Blue Cross for hospital, and Blue Shield for doctor's expenses. Interactions with physicians and with local hospitals were very personal and vastly different than they are today.

Today, we see the consequence of these experiences and exposures as a greater disease burden of respiratory ailments, renal disease, thyroid disease, and blood diseases than we hope will develop in later generations. In addition, today's older people are at a severe disadvantage negotiating today's health-care system and computer-driven bureaucracy and paperwork. They did not grow up in a world of computers and health-insurance companies. But many younger people have a romantic belief that life was better in the "old days." The truth is that we now live much longer, have better diets, fresher food, safer living and working conditions, and more free time to exercise and enjoy life than ever before.

Having lived for several decades, older people can say, "Been there; saw that; done that!" They may look with reserved tolerance and amusement at the rat race they see going on around them—but do not want to get involved. Like parents who realize their children don't always accept or even want their advice, they remain silent, watching younger people learn things the hard way—by themselves. Older people may feel tired and more insecure about their capacity to make a difference. They may sense the futility or folly of getting actively involved in the same kinds of fights and issues they did when they were younger, and are now too exhausted or burnt out to get involved again. Fads, community concerns, economic problems, and political issues all have a way of cycling and coming back again and again with only slightly different variations. Having gone around these cycles before, older people usually have a very different perspective of these issues than do younger people.

A very frightening consequence of this change in past experiences seems to be an observed age-dependent difference in attitude regarding the importance of immunizations. Younger people, with no personal history of infectious diseases such as polio, hepatitis, diphtheria, tetanus, whooping cough, pneumococcal pneumonia, shingles, or flu pandemics, seem much more complacent about these illnesses and seem hesitant in accepting the vaccinations recommended by our leading health authorities. This is even evident in younger health professionals themselves. Parents are hesitant to have their children immunized, but usually succumb to the pressure of school regulations. We are now at increasing risk of seeing a resurgence of some of these diseases that younger doctors have never encountered, nor might not even recognize.

A lesson for younger people who try to teach older people is that they may instead be able to learn from the older person;

they should also realize that they might first have to prove themselves to older individuals. They may appear a lot younger than the older people's children or grandchildren, and therefore need to demonstrate they know what they are talking about.

How fast do we age?

We all recognize that different animal species have different life expectancies and rates of aging (consider the tortoise and elephant compared to a bee or a fruit fly). Between inbred mouse strains, whose members are genetically identical, there are great differences in longevity. Using these inbred mouse strains, one can identify "aging genes." And within our own human species, there appear to be genes that seem to control the rate of aging. Some individuals and their family members appear much younger and energetic than their peers. If one looks at family photos, they always seemed younger than others around them. Other families seem to age more rapidly than expected. This supports the belief that there are "longevity genes." Current research is examining how exactly these genes exert their effect. There are some medical conditions in which there is "premature" and rapid aging with a much-reduced life expectancy. Illness seems to hasten the aging process.

As we age, differences between people increase. In the developing newborn, it is easy to anticipate their expected maturation: when they will smile, walk, talk, and grow teeth. Individual differences increase as we age (some caused by disease and lifestyle, but others by the expanding inherent differences between individuals). This makes it much more difficult to predict an older person's "biologic" age, or to extrapolate and generalize about all older people. Inter-individual heterogeneity is one of the hallmarks of aging, and makes generalizations about aging less reliable. This point should be kept in mind throughout reading this book. Older people are not all the same, nor do they age at the same rate or in the same way. Since we can't alter our genes, the best we can do to retard aging is to remain as healthy as we can.

How important is greater longevity?

Regardless of our views and feelings about aging, we know that we will age, and that we all will die. People have been searching for the "Elixir of life" or the Fountain of Youth for millennia. Is this really what we want for ourselves—to live forever and never die? World population is already reaching a foreseeable limit where our food and water supply, as well as adequate living space, would not be able to sustain the population. Experiments with rodents show that overcrowding leads to diminished procreation, and animals killing each other (the Malthusian phenomenon).

The goal of science and medicine perhaps should be one promoted by one of my mentors—Lewis Thomas. Everyone should live well till some undetermined, natural programmed age, when suddenly every cell in our body loses its capacity to sustain itself, and we crumble into a heap of dust—no suffering or aging, but instead living well till some moment when we quickly crumble and die.

Human life expectancy has expanded markedly over the past century. Notwithstanding the stories of Methuselah, Abraham, and Moses, life expectancy in Biblical times was estimated to have been thirty-five to forty years of age. Nature and natural selection would have an interest in keeping us alive only till our children could survive, procreate, and maintain our species. Otto von Bismarck, as chancellor of Germany at the end of the nineteenth century, set the age of sixty-five as the age citizens became "old" and could expect public support. Since in the nineteenth century, life expectancy was sixty to sixty-five, he wasn't giving too much away. But the age of sixty-five has persisted in most societies as a defining age. Today, life expectancy extends into the eighties, and we talk about the aged as being over eighty-five, and, in some areas, over ninety.

The fear of aging is usually associated with the fear of disease. Aged individuals are frequently viewed or imagined as being ill or incapacitated one way or another. The very word *senile*, meaning "old," was reinterpreted as meaning "demented." However, we regularly see individuals in their nineties in our community who appear physically well, and who seem intellectually and functionally intact and self-sufficient. Many are still working productively. We are not surprised to meet someone over one hundred. Aging itself does not necessarily mean infirmity. But health becomes more fragile. Mostly it seems it is disease, rather than aging that causes debility.

Females, on the average, live 5–10 percent longer than males in every mammalian species studied. Hormonal activity seems to be responsible for some of this difference. Castrate a newborn male mouse, and it will live as long as the newborn female. Begin injecting the female mouse with male hormones, and it will die earlier. With longer life expectancies, and normally marrying men several years older than themselves, it is no surprise why there are so many more widows than widowers. Severe protein and caloric restriction at a young age can also lengthen our years. Reducing the calories and protein intake for years seems to enable all mammals to live longer (although they usually become sterile, and may not be very happy). This then impacts on what will be discussed below: Is it our goal to live longer, or to live happier?

How do we age?

But we do age—despite how very much we may object to this reality. One of nature's rules is that we cannot keep

14

sixteen-year-old parts more than one year of our life. Further, our goal should not be to die with sixteen-year-old parts. We easily see the visible signs of aging in our hair, our eyes, teeth, and skin. But every organ is aging: our bones, arteries, joints, our vision, our hearing, and bladder. Our ligaments and tendons stiffen and we become stiffer. At the cellular level, we also are aging. Indeed, we cannot halt the aging of any organ, no matter how we may try, even with surgery and cosmetics. Not only do our structures age, but every bodily function and system also age, including our immune system and defenses against infection. We may try to look younger, but we delude ourselves when we think we can remain young.

One of the most startling aspects of aging is the loss of height. People are shocked when they measure their height and realize how many inches they have lost. Most of this loss is due to the inexorable drying of cartilage. This is the cartilage that makes up our intervertebral disks, the cartilage in our hips, knees, and ankles, which had served as "spacers" and natural shock absorbers in our spine and joints. As cartilage dries, we lose height and the shock absorbency that used to be the role of healthy cartilage. (More about this will be discussed in the section on back pain). We begin the process of joint trauma and arthritis. We don't realize this loss of height, since everyone around us is losing height at nearly the same rate. Although some of the height loss may be due to posture, or curvature of the spine (scoliosis and kyphosis), much of it is due to cartilage volume loss. Most of us also gain weight with aging. We also look fatter, since we are cramming our weight into a shorter package. Because of the intense concern about weight and appearance, many patients get very upset when they weigh more at the doctor's office than they do at home, and usually blame the doctor's scale. They need reminding that when they weigh themselves at home, it is usually first thing in the morning, after going to the toilet. Their stomachs are empty, their bladder is empty, their colon is empty, and they have not yet accumulated any fluid in their feet. This is a naked, baseline weight. After eating, dressing, and drinking, how can they expect a weight later in the day to be as low as the one measured at home? Also, our metabolism slows, and physical activities usually diminish with aging—but we still can eat, and get considerable pleasure from food. No small wonder why we gain weight.

But our "souls" or mind, although also aging, still seems to function as it always did, at least to the individual involved. We are not aware of our brain's aging unless a new neurologic event occurs. There are clear neurologic changes that can be measured with aging: Reflexes and reaction times slow. The mind is not as "fast" as it used to be, and a mild cognitive impairment of aging (MCI) occurs commonly. (More about this will be discussed in a later section on memory.) This is often expressed as forgetting for the moment where the keys are, or was the door locked, or what was the name of that person to whom we were just introduced? We may fumble for a word or name that pops back into our mind hours later. If distracted, we may forget for the moment what we were just saying or doing. These changes can frighten the individual and their family into believing this represents the onset of dementia. These issues, however, can occur in very well functioning individuals, and usually do not disturb those who feel reasonably secure in their capacities. Healthy older persons may still function as they did twenty to thirty years previously.

We have a reasonably good idea of what it is to be young, as all of us have at one time been young. The same is not true of being "old," and we often speculate about what an older person feels or needs. This can backfire in several ways. A person with disease may attribute their complaints to "simply getting old" and defer seeking medical attention. Many may have developed their own home-remedy way of treating any symptom and will try this first. It is far cheaper and easier to try a home-remedy than to see a doctor and run the risk of extensive testing and hospitalization (see below). Others may see every complaint as a symptom of some impending calamity. These uncertainties can have significant ramifications. If symptoms bother an individual, it is best to explore their cause with someone who has greater experience in dealing with such problems, such as their doctor. Not having firsthand experience with being older can lead to other problems. Programs intended for "senior citizens" are usually made by much younger individuals, who only project and suppose what older people might enjoy, need, or how they might like to be treated. Contrary to a popular belief of younger people, individuals at sixty-five years of age do not suddenly develop a passion for playing Bingo! Older people also object to being patronized, or being treated as if they were deaf, demented, or infantile. Regardless of what they may have achieved in their working lives, older people usually resent being called "pop" or "dear." They may resent being yelled at just because they are old and therefore considered deaf. Marketing people recognize that the elderly live, travel, vote, take educational courses, shop, and enjoy life's bounties. They may have more disposable income than do many younger individuals, and thus can be a strong economic force in the community. Much advertising is directed at the elderly.

Having lived a long time, older people have lived through depressions and repeated financial crises. They are usually retired from work and living on fixed pensions, retirement plans, savings, and social security, with little expectation of their incomes going up significantly. For some, the combined income may make them more financially secure than at any previous time of their life. Others may face added financial worries. They may feel the financial needs of their children and grandchildren and want to help them or leave them an inheritance. Some elderly may feel that retaining their wealth provides them with greater security, respect, influence, independence, and power as they age and subsequently are afraid of losing this wealth. A common goal and dream of older immigrants was to work hard, "make it" in America, and leave something behind for their children (who shouldn't have to work so hard). With rising prices, taxes, interest rates, etc., many older people often have to ration their spending, and the dream of leaving something behind for their children evaporates. Medical care and purchasing medicines now often competes with other basic needs. As discussed below, insurance plans, free community facilities, and pharmaceutical programs for the needy can help, but elderly people have their pride and may not take advantage of these programs.

How our body composition changes with age

With aging, there are some very definite changes that occur in our bodies. Aside from what we see in the mirror, with graying hair, yellowing teeth, wrinkling skin, there are some very significant changes occurring in our general body composition. Lean body mass (or muscle mass) decreases; muscle tone generally also decreases. Total fat increases and total body water decreases. Flexible tissue becomes stiffer due to changes in fibrous tissue and collagen. These changes are not trivial, and are very important for doctors to recognize, because many of the commonly taken medications will have altered distribution in our bodies (as compared to younger individuals') as a result of these changes in body composition. Elimination of medicines can also be slowed by reduction in the capacity of our kidneys and liver to eliminate the medicines as we age. This means that medications in the amounts and doses that we had been taking for many years might work differently as we get older.

Regarding specific organs, our chest wall (or thorax) is stiffer, and we can't breathe as deeply as we once did. Our heart muscle is stiffer, and can't relax as well to allow the same blood filling as when we were younger. Indeed, the function of every organ is somewhat compromised with aging. But, since we were born with so much reserve function, in the absence of disease, we should have more than enough function in all our vital organs for survival to a very old age.

How the Elderly Are Viewed—Common Stereotypes

In a common stereotype, older people are viewed as being somewhat cognitively impaired, unkempt, always cold, wearing moth-eaten, thread-bare sweaters, wearing stained and soiled old clothes, having bad body odor (including the smell of urine or stool), being hard of hearing, and generally being feeble. But, on the positive side, they also are perceived as being good-wishing and pleasant.

Some of this stereotype has a valid basis. As discussed in greater detail below, older people often have less visual acuity than younger people: they don't see the stains and holes in their clothes as well as can their children; their sense of smell is usually diminished. There may be difficulty in controlling their urine and bowels. Children, seeing the problem, frequently try unsuccessfully to get their parents to buy new clothes or wash more often. Older people have a fear of slipping and falling in the bathtub. As a result, if living alone, they often don't bathe and wash (or shave) as frequently as they did when they were not living alone. With less subcutaneous fat they have less insulation. Their slower metabolism and decreased muscle mass means less heat being generated, and they feel the cold more acutely than their children, which is why they keep their homes overheated and may wear sweaters even in the hot summer. With depression, and nowhere to go, they are often less concerned with their physical appearance. Shopping, going to the beauty parlor, and having their clothes cleaned professionally and frequently requires more effort, and carries a significant price tag; older people who may be financially insecure may hesitate in doing things that will cost the extra money. It may take more effort and expense, but it is important that the older person make the effort to appear neat, clean, and well groomed. This maintains their standing among their family, neighbors, and friends, and gives them more dignity.

There still is significant ageism (age discrimination) in our society. *Ageism*, a word coined by Robert Butler fifty years ago, generally refers to discrimination against the elderly; it is based on a perceived negative stereotype and reflects negative attitudes regarding the elderly in regard to their performance, abilities, or competence. Lumping any group of people based on a single attribute may be convenient at times but will always be uneven, probably prejudicial, and usually unfair. Since advancing age is associated with the greatest inter-individual variability of any age group, stereotyping the elderly is even more inappropriate than for younger individuals.

Ageism is seen among the elderly themselves, who may attribute every complaint they experience to "getting old." They may even complain about their friends and peers who seem to be getting "old so fast," while they don't recognize that it is an illness, and not aging, that is responsible for the changes. Denying one's own age is another form of ageism. Ageism is also manifested, unfortunately, in the way many doctors ascribe the patient's complaints to their age, before fully investigating other possible causes for their complaints. This can have tragic consequences. Ageism is often manifested in hiring applicants for a job, when an older person is refused insurance or denied the opportunity to rent a car based solely on their age. Since "ageism" implies the special treatment of an individual based entirely on their advanced age, the flip side of "ageism" is rewarding an individual, not by merit or need, but solely on the basis of their age. This is evident in the "senior" discounts at theaters or museums. Like any other characteristic of an individual (e.g., race, religion, ethnicity, gender, sexual preference), advanced age should not be the sole criterion used to discriminate against or to favor an individual. Function, merit, or need would be preferable and more appropriate criteria.

People frequently insert the word *old* into describing an individual as if that were an important adjective. "Stupid old man!"; "Little old lady!" How would we react if we inserted a descriptive term of religion or race instead of "old"? We would probably find that objectionable, as it is irrelevant, and is likely being used with derogatory intent. The adjective *old* is not, nor should be, the central issue; it focuses on age as the most important variable—and that itself is ageism.

There is no consistent way in how to describe older individuals in the most "politically correct" or "pc" way. Terms like "elderly", "aged", "aging", "senior", "old", and "geriatric", all have slightly different connotations, although none are pejorative; adding an adjective such as "very" adds an extra dimension to how much older the person may be, but is still a subjective evaluation.

What Should Be Our Goals of Living?

So we are faced with the reality that we must age. But what is the goal or purpose of our life? Is it to die young? Is it to die with sixteen-year-old parts? Is it even to die healthy, or with the best cholesterol, the lowest weight, the best figure, or the best arteries? Is the goal of life to die rich or with a maximum of possessions?

I would suggest that the goal of living should be in living the best life one can—living to achieve the most satisfaction as we possibly can—both with quality and longevity. I believe there are four essential elements needed to fully enjoy a good life (the *4Ls of Living*): LIVING (and trying to get the most satisfaction that one can obtain in life); LEARNING (continued learning, keeping an inquisitive mind and enlarging one's knowledge and wisdom), LOVING (family and friends; being socially involved, not isolated), and LAUGHING (enjoying the humor that abounds about us). This doesn't mean we should live hedonistic lifestyles, living only for our sole immediate gratification and for momentary pleasure. We must continue to plan for the future, but we shouldn't put off living either. Also, humans are social animals, and our behavior must be weighed in the context of the impact that what we do can have on others around us—not only on our family and those we love, but also on society in general. Our own enjoyment of life depends to a large extent upon how others regard and treat us. Our lives are short enough, and the future is always uncertain—we should make the most of our lives while we can.

We usually know what is best for us. In medicine, as in life, our decisions are based on the expectation of the benefit or value to us as a whole vs. the expected penalty or risk. There are risks inherent in living. There are risks taken when flying in airplanes, driving on highways, taking taxis in busy cities, crossing streets, etc. If we are afraid to take risks, we are afraid to live, and we lose much of the value of our lives. Would any of us want to spend our entire life confined to a safe, padded windowless room, so as to avoid the risks and dangers of the outside world? Indeed, living requires our taking risks. I don't believe any doctor ever recommended a patient begin skydiving, bungee jumping, mountain climbing, or sports car racing for medical reasons. But people do these things. We live our lives to do things we enjoy, understanding the benefits and the risks of our actions. No one can tell us which risks we find worth taking, nor can anyone tell us the value we place on any planned activity. We are the best judges of how we feel, and of what action we believe would have the most beneficial impact on our lives. We may, and often do, make mistakes. Everyone is entitled to make his or her own mistakes. Our expectations do not always materialize the way we had expected: sometimes things turn out much better than we had anticipated, sometimes much worse. Sometimes the penalty turns out to be much worse than we expected, sometimes not nearly as bad as we had feared. We never know the results for certain before the fact. And we can never totally avoid taking risks. There are no guarantees in life.

In medicine, the same rules apply. When we take medications or undergo tests or procedures we weigh benefit and risk. What will be the benefit to us, and what will be the risk or penalty of any particular action (or any alternative action, for that matter)? Both sides of the issue need to be evaluated. If a medicine does no good, or has no benefit, why should we take it? If a medicine makes us ill, or costs too much, it might not be worth taking. What we all want is the medicine or procedure that gives us the maximal benefit for the least penalty. If there is a cheaper medicine with the same benefit, why should we not take it? If a procedure with less of a risk can accomplish the same goal, why should we not try that procedure first?

Making Priorities and Life Choices for Healthy Living

An extremely important component of successful aging is realizing what is truly important, and what is not, in a person's life. People need to reflect upon what problems bother them the most, and then make decisions about priorities and other life choices. This is true with all our medical conditions. Often the older person becomes overwhelmed with the stresses of aging. Too many things are going wrong, and too many doctors are recommending different treatments. After running from doctor to doctor, a person can get tired and depressed. Too much seems to be going wrong too quickly. Their bodies seem to be falling apart. There is a risk that the older person will just give up and do nothing. The truth simply is that ALL the organs are older, but not all problems need to be treated. A minor blemish might be considered a horrible affliction by a young competitive person but be totally ignored by an older person. The priority and need for attention does not reside in the condition, but rather in its impact and how it disturbs the person's life. What is needed is some prioritization of each complaint—working with the doctor to understand the significance of each problem.

If we ask the older patient what is it that they really want out of life, as they get older, or what they fear most about aging, we get common answers. "We do no want to become a burden on our children or grandchildren." They fear a loss of autonomy and independence. They also fear being in chronic pain. Looking at aging from this perspective (what it is that disturbs the older person the most), patients and their doctors can focus their attention on what measures would really make an improvement in the person's life.

Aspects of independent functioning are commonly grouped into ADLs (activities of daily living) and IADLs (instrumental activities of daily living). ADLs include standing, walking, sitting up, getting out of bed, self-feeding and -drinking, toileting, washing and grooming, and dressing and undressing. IADLs include telephoning, performing housework, taking medications, managing money and finances, shopping, driving, and using transportation. If any of these key functions of living are compromised, the individual will need additional help. I would argue that the two highest priorities should be (1) enjoying some aspect (or aspects) of life, and (2) not being in pain.

Functionally, I stress that anything that can be done to maximize the quality of living should be of primary concern. These include problems with vision, hearing, ambulation and moving, and bladder and bowel control.

Since each of us is different, and each of us has different fears and conditions, each person ranks what bothers them the most. We are bombarded with advertising that addresses some medical condition for which some company is offering a remedy, as if that condition needs immediate attention. What I have recommended to my patients is that they think about how their life would be, if that condition were not an immediate problem. Ranking and placing priority is best accomplished by considering which specific condition, if addressed, would improve a person's life the most (assuming there is a therapy available that could resolve or control the bothersome condition). (More about this is presented in section III on doctor/patient interactions).

To enjoy life maximally, some functions or conditions seem more important for quality of life than others (even when there's no threat to life). Pain, for example, is a no-no. It is hard to enjoy life while one is in pain. Relief of pain is a priority for the patient, and relief of suffering should be a priority for the physician. Unfortunately, chronic pain usually results in need for chronic painkillers—a condition by which the victim of pain is sometimes cast and viewed as a manipulator and seeker of strong analgesics (i.e., narcotics). However, chronic use of narcotics does lead to dependency and addiction.

Being able to see is another top priority. Life can never be as rewarding when a person can't see as when he or she can. Hearing similarly can provide much pleasure in life: hearing one's loved ones, hearing music, and hearing the sounds of nature. Mobility and independence rank up there with important functions. Vision, hearing, and mobility are also safety issues. Loss of control of one's eliminations is very disturbing, and limits the activities that a person might want to do. An unpleasant odor will keep family and friends at a distance. And lastly, depression robs the individual of the most valuable asset anyone possesses: the ability to enjoy one's life.

Surprisingly, the geriatrician faces an uphill battle with the patient in tackling many of these problems. Too often, the older individual accepts problems in the above categories. Surprisingly, they often focus all their medical attention on their circulation, their heart, their fear of cancer, fear of a stroke, a failing memory, or their bone density, even when these conditions do not immediately affect their daily function and enjoyment of life, and would probably not cause their demise for many, many years.

Pain is one of those conditions that cannot be independently or objectively assessed. As a practical measure, the individual with pain should note how the pain interferes with their normal life, its character (sharp, dull, piercing, throbbing, or shooting), and its location in the body. The intensity of pain is generally given by its status on a scale of one to ten, where one is barely noticeable and ten is excruciating. The duration and frequency of the pain is also an important feature, as is whether it is a new or recurrent pain. And lastly, the individual should make note of what they have found, if anything, that makes the pain less, and what they feel brings it on or makes it worse (such as changes in position, activity, eating, or toileting). Presenting this information to your doctor can be immensely helpful for diagnosing the cause of the pain, as well as developing a strategy to reduce the pain.

Satisfactory management of chronic pain can be very frustrating for the patient, the patient's family and friends, and the physicians caring for the individual. People vary tremendously in their pain thresholds or willingness to talk about their pain. Taking pain medication alone may bypass the more difficult question of why the person is having pain. Pain can be seen with inflammation, with vascular insufficiency, tumors, nerve inflammation, or psychosomatically. There is always a cause for the *complaint* of pain, but it can be hard to elucidate. When the complaint of pain is chronic and its cause has eluded diagnosis, many doctors and family members may feel that the individual is trying to manipulate the family, or is seeking narcotics to satisfy an addiction. Even the patient himself may begin to question why he is having pain. A psychological or psychiatric evaluation is often helpful in understanding the significance of the complaint. Chronic pain is always very disturbing and frustrating for the family, individual, and doctor. Sometimes it needs a fresh look by someone who comes to the problem with no "baggage" and studies the history, the test results, and the physical findings with a new perspective. Taking narcotics by pill or by injection is a valuable therapy in patients with chronic severe pain, but carries the risk and stigma of dependency and addiction. Taking too many narcotic medications runs the risk of having the person becoming unsteady, falling, and fracturing bones; too little analgesic, and the person is suffering for no particularly important purpose. Physicians who specialize in pain management are becoming more numerous throughout the country.

There are many types of therapies that are available and can be tried before resorting to narcotics: physical therapy, exercise, non-narcotic medicines, injections of steroids and anesthetics, braces and supports, TENS (trans-epidermal nerve stimulator), massage, acupuncture, and hypnosis usually carry less risk to the patient than do narcotics. It is a priority to understand the cause of the pain, and to develop a strategy for unraveling its cause and how best to deal with the problem.

Visual disturbances are major problems that affect the quality of life. All older individuals should regularly see their ophthalmologist. If the individual has diabetes, hypertension, or vascular disease, the frequency of eye exams should be increased. When they have trouble seeing, older patients seek help from ophthalmologists fairly quickly. The suggestion of wearing corrective lenses rarely disturbs the patient, but recommendations of surgery, intraocular injections, or laser therapies can meet some hesitation. Stiffening and opacification of the lenses in the eyes occurs in everyone as they age, and progresses throughout their lives. As a cataract becomes denser, it produces problems with experiencing glare in bright light, seeing haloes around lights, difficulty focusing (having a more rigid and less flexible lens), and having reduced vision in dim light due to less light penetrating the more opaque lens. Of all surgeries performed, cataract surgery is the most common, and is considered the surgery with the greatest patient satisfaction, although complications can occur, as they can with any surgical procedure. Other eye problems associated with aging are "dry eyes" (discussed below), glaucoma (too much pressure within the eye, threatening the vision), and macular degeneration. The macula is the portion of the retina on which we focus the image, and is the area of our sharpest color vision. Causes for macular degeneration (which can be accompanied by bleeding [wet] or nonbleeding [dry]), although unknown, seem to involve our focusing all radiation on our macula. As with focusing light onto a single spot on paper with a magnifying glass, and producing enough heat to start a fire, the focusing of light and radiation on the macula can cause localized damage to this area. Why only some people develop macular degeneration suggests there may be individual defects in the protective and repair mechanisms in those people who do develop it. Therapy for macular degeneration today includes antioxidant vitamins for dry, and injections to retard blood vessel growth directly into the eye for wet. Older people should receive regular eye examinations by an ophthalmologist.

Hearing issues pose a larger problem for everyone involved with the elderly person. Older people with hearing problems usually do not complain about hearing loss, and may try to deny or hide it. They rarely rush to the audiologist or their doctor. Affected people usually complain that everyone around them is "mumbling more." The family complains to the doctor that the hearing problem is driving everyone in the family crazy. One unfortunate scenario is that the older person with a hearing loss just raises the sound volume of the TV, CD player, or radio. They may not hear the banging on the walls, ceiling, or floor caused by their angry neighbors who are bothered by the noise. That individual can lose the good wishes of everyone sharing their building, and can't understand why neighbors have become so unfriendly. This can lead to isolation and depression.

The cost of hearing aids, their appearance, and the fine motor skills needed to insert them and change the batteries may present a hardship to some people. As a result, older people with hearing issues usually claim that they can hear well enough if only others around them would speak more clearly and not mumble, and that the hearing aid is not cost-efficient. Indeed, in a quiet room with no ambient noise, the individual might hear quite adequately, but in a car, a restaurant, a function hall, or a crowded family get-together, the hearing "goes." I remind this person that it is in these latter settings, when they are with the people they love most, that hearing is most important. If they cannot hear and answer their grandchildren and great-grandchildren, there is a good possibility that these children will stop talking to their elderly relative. The cause for the hearing loss may be as simple as impacted earwax in the ear canals, and clearing out the wax can make a dramatic improvement in hearing. Other times it is due to a problem with the small bones in the middle ear that transmit the sound from the eardrum to the inner ear, where the vibrations of the sound are converted to nerve messages in the cochlea and transmitted to the brain. Cochlear implants are now being done more frequently for individuals who have "nerve deafness."

Poor control of bladder and bowel function affects millions of older people, and can have far-reaching consequences. To reduce the severity of the problem, afflicted people often restrict their intake of fluids and become significantly dehydrated (discussed below), and they often stop taking any needed diuretic, blaming the medicine for their problem. Voiding problems are always an embarrassment to those with the problem and those close to them. In men, their prostates enlarge throughout their life, due to continued growth stimulation by testosterone. The prostate surrounds the urethra (the duct that carries urine to the outside), and as the prostate enlarges, it can block the egress of urine, like pinching the neck of a filled balloon stops the air from leaving (see Fig. 7, p. 136). In older women, postmenopausal changes and changes caused by past pregnancies and deliveries can result in relaxation of the pelvic floor and a "dropped" bladder. These often lead to problems of urinary control. The urge to urinate occurs when the bladder muscle "twitches" and sends an impulse to the brain. The twitch occurs when the pressure in the bladder reaches some specific level, which varies between individuals. If there is an obstruction as the bladder empties and the pressure within the bladder drops (like air going out of a tire), there may not be enough pressure to totally empty the organ. When there is not enough pressure left within the bladder to push all the remaining urine past the obstruction, the urination dribbles to a stop. If a considerable volume of urine is left in the bladder, it won't take much more urine being added to have the volume, pressure, and twitch occurring a very short time later. This causes increased frequency and urgency of urination. In other persons, the bladder may be irritable or overactive. It seems to be in a state of spasm, where the accumulation of minimal amounts of additional urine increases the pressure to the twitch point and a need to void. Some common medicines cause the bladder to relax too much, so that the bladder lacks the pressure to expel the urine. These medicines include many over-the-counter medications used for allergy and sleep. This is one of the most common causes of the very disturbing inability to urinate, or leaking urine without control.

Urinary incontinence is both embarrassing and uncomfortable. Sometimes, neurological problems affect bladder function so that the bladder cannot properly empty. These are called neurogenic bladder disorders. In these cases, a permanent catheter may be necessary. Urinary tract infections can irritate the bladder and make it less efficient as a urine storage container. In these conditions, the person always seems to have a need to urinate. They are continually running to the bathroom, and this disturbs their life, both while awake and while asleep. Patients should realize that the problem is in the bladder control, not the kidney. Patients frequently confuse the functions of the kidney and the bladder: the kidney filters and regulates the blood while making urine, while the bladder stores the urine. People can get into significant health problems if they stop taking a prescribed diuretic. This is particularly unfortunate, since the problem lies in the bladder, and not the kidney. They need to discuss this with their doctor.

Treatments for voiding problems may include wearing an absorbent "shield" or undergarment. Exercise of the muscles that control continence is very helpful if the person is motivated enough to exercise these muscles regularly. In these exercises, called *Kegel* exercises, the person contracts the muscles that hold back urination for twenty to thirty seconds, and then relaxes them. This is repeated twenty to thirty times each exercise period, which should be done several times a day. Medicines can relax the bladder, if it is spastic. Surgeries and injections of collagen and Botox can help restore continence. Surgical options in women include several types of procedures to "hold up" the dropped bladder. Urologists and gynecologists can discuss the various options available. In men with enlarging prostates, there are medicines that can relax the prostate and urethra, and others that shrink the prostate. If medicines fail, there are several options to open the channel, which the prostate is compressing. With the advent of lasers and newer technologies, the old surgery of "Roto-Rooter" cutting is now rarely performed. In some men, the wearing of a condom catheter that is connected to a leg-bag allows the man to urinate at will without any spillage, odor, or embarrassment. With a condom catheter, the urinary tube extends from the condom and does not penetrate into the bladder. Unlike an indwelling Foley catheter, the condom catheter can be removed and applied without difficulty or need for sterility, but it does not traverse the prostate, and cannot be used to manage the obstruction caused by prostatic enlargement. When all else fails, there are adult absorbent "diapers" that many individuals use. They are readily available over the counter in pharmacies, and are designed for both men and women.

A common problem seen in the elderly is dehydration (as mentioned above). With aging, the sensation of thirst is diminished. One rarely sees older people walking in the street carrying bottles of water. Since many older people have urinary control problems, including the need to get up frequently at night to urinate, or getting to the toilet quickly enough to avoid an accident, an easy solution quickly discovered is to limit the fluid intake. If you drink less, you will pee less. This works for a while, but imposes the penalty of dehydration if carried out for a long period. Dehydration is not good for the circulation, for the bowel (where stool can desiccate and become dry, "like a rock"). Dehydration is not good for the kidney, the skin, the brain, the lungs, or any organ that requires good circulation. Respiratory secretions thicken, and are harder to expectorate. It is as if the person was sacrificing all of his or her organs on the altar of the bladder. It is a bad bargain. Studies have shown that the average aged patient admitted to the hospital is significantly dehydrated and needs liters of intravenous fluid just to correct the fluid imbalance. Limiting fluids or stopping diuretics should never be the way to treat bladder and urination problems.

Fatigue, weakness, and mobility issues are another class of important problems in the elderly that affect quality of life. There are many causes for excessive fatigue and mobility disorders: depression, arthritis, and neurological conditions of balance, weakness, and foot disorders. Strength and balance can be improved by exercise. Stretching is helpful to reduce stiffness. Many older individuals with weakness and fatigue rest more. However, strength does not increase with rest. Any athletic person knows that it is not rest but exercise that improves strength. For people who had led an active life, the thought of exercise is not anathema, but for couch potatoes, exercise is usually not an option easily accepted or continued for any meaningful duration. Exercising with another individual makes exercise a social encounter, and may make it more acceptable. Consultation with physiatrists (rehab doctors), neurologists, podiatrists, and therapists may all be helpful in developing a strategy to improve mobility and flexibility.

Independent living is an important goal of most people. Simple issues like bathing, dressing, preparing food, getting out of a chair may pose problems. Having a person in the house to help is often met with fierce resistance. Children often become frustrated and infuriated trying to convince their parent to accept an aide. An aide is viewed as a direct threat to the older person's sense of independence and self-sufficiency. Also there is the problem of expense. People are reluctant to jump into the expense of paying for a caretaker or home attendant. This can be an open-ended expense, with no clear total cost envisioned. The reality is, however, that when individuals lose so much function that they are essentially helpless and need assistance with most of their daily activities, life expectancy is no longer measured in decades or multiple years, and families might want the last several years of a loved one's life to be less stressful and have them better cared for.

There is a lot of room for negotiation. One can hire an attendant for as little as a few hours a day for several days a week, or up to twenty-four hours every day. One can have an attendant for food preparation, cleaning, shopping, and accompanying the older person on scheduled appointments, going to a movie, or for more extensive personal care such as dressing, washing, eating, and toileting. Having another person in the home carries the risk that the attendant might try to impose their wishes and decisions on the older person. But if one attendant does not work out well, the need may still be valid, and the answer might be to replace the attendant. A good agency or a reliable case manager will get well-screened, honest attendants (and replacements if the attendant is unable to come one day). Despite the initial resistance, most older people who need additional help accept the idea of having "help at home" once they experience it, and realize their fears were not as great as expected, and the rewards were significantly greater.

In our society we also recognize the reality of personal physical and verbal abuse by a person in power against another who is defenseless. We are all familiar with stories of child abuse. However, there is also elder abuse caused by spouses, children, and attendants. Whenever individuals are vulnerable and cannot express themselves clearly or fight back, they are at risk from abuse by angry and frustrated individuals. It is very hard to know whether bruises seen on an older demented person were caused by imbalance and falling, or by intentional attack. Accusing an individual of intentionally hurting a loved one is extremely difficult, and one would need absolute proof of the offense. Unfortunately many older people complain of being mistreated, when the other person is merely trying to help them. They also can have bruises and black-and-blue marks caused by their medicines, the fragility of their skin, and their imbalance. People are beginning to use the mini-cam to "spy" on happenings when their children, and now their parents, are being cared for by a nanny or an attendant; abuse does sometimes occur, and can come from almost anyone.

What we see is that there are lifestyle choices that need to be made—choices in where the older person should live. Many older people do not want to be a burden on their family. Some are too proud to accept help- financial or physical. What are the medical problems that really need immediate attention? Again, it is an issue of priorities. The problems associated with aging will only get worse when the individual gets sick. Most of the problems encountered with advanced age are neither new nor unique; many other individuals who have come before have dealt with similar problems. While the problems may be new to a particular person, they are not new problems to those who deal frequently with issues of this kind. There are many service agencies in the community that can help explain the choices and guide family members through the difficult decisions.

Healthy living in old age requires some amount of planning and realistic thinking, and is discussed further in a later section (section III).

SECTION II — ILLNESS AND HEALTH

Aging seems to be the only available way to live a long life -

DANIEL FRANCOIS ESPRIT AUBER

Medical Problems Associated with Aging

Many of the medical problems an older person faces are merely extensions of the types of problems they faced when they were younger. Older individuals have already had experience dealing with complaints they had before, and may feel comfortable in managing their own care. However, many conditions and complaints are new, clearly age-related, present differently, or have added complications and implications that make them more complex in the elderly. Aging adds another level of complexity to all medical conditions. Unlike younger individuals, where a complaint generally can be ascribed to a single disorder, in older people, with age-related problems affecting all their organs, complaints are often due to a complex blend or interaction of several disorders. The challenge in geriatrics is to determine the relative contributions of *all* the conditions that may be contributing to the complaint. Successfully managing a condition that is a major contributing factor can result in major improvement in the patient's general condition. Treatment of a minor contributing condition might have little benefit.

Described below are the problems and complaints associated with common diseases that I have observed most frequently and repeatedly, and for which my patients were seeking understanding: a simple explanation of what might be going on, and how patients (the older patient or the caregiver) might think about the issue.

What You Should Know About Illness and Hospitalization

"I don't feel well and I'm afraid!" Illness happens, and happens more often in the elderly. When older individuals feel sick, many thoughts flash through their minds: "Is this IT—THE END?" Many old and recurrent fears merge and emerge. If people live alone, it's worse. They might like to deny they're feeling badly, and may hope the feeling goes away by itself—but it usually doesn't.

Probably the older person's biggest fear is that they will end up in the hospital. If they call their children, their family will worry about them, and if they call the doctor, they may be taken to the hospital, even against their will. Just being a patient in an emergency room itself is an ordeal they all dread. How long will they lie there in an uncomfortable state before being admitted to a room or taken for surgery? Too many old friends, relatives, and peers had gone to the hospital and never came home. They had ended up dying, or going to nursing homes. Will this now happen to them?

As a practical answer, they should consult the doctor they trust. If their doctor is unavailable (and is being covered by an unknown doctor), they still should get professional advice.

Recognize, however, that this may be a two-way problem: not only may they not know the covering doctor, but also the covering doctor may not know them. When any physician does not know the patient sufficiently well, there is a tendency to be overly cautious. This may be translated into referral to the emergency department of the closest hospital, and ordering more tests and consultations than would have been ordered by a doctor more familiar with a patient's medical history. Things may not be as bad as older patients fear, even if they do end up receiving a lot of emergency medical attention.

Hospitalization represents a major threat to their very way of life. In the hospital, they know they will lose their independence and will no longer control what's happening to them. Strangers begin making decisions regarding what they should do, how they should live, how they must spend their precious recourses. They don't understand the hospital routine, or how and why things are being done to them. If there is a language problem, it gets worse. Do people really understand what it is they're trying to say? Are there cultural differences that are not understood or respected? They don't feel well, and people keep asking them the same questions, prodding them, sticking needles into them, and sending them around the hospital for uncomfortable and often frightening tests. There is an accompanying loss of dignity, modesty, self-respect, and individual identity. Running through their minds is also the issue of major expenses. How well will their insurance cover the costs of the hospital stay? How much of the bill will be their responsibility?

If they do end up going to the emergency department, will they be admitted? Will they be sent home in the middle of the night? What should they bring with them: their medicines, a toothbrush, their address book, cash, mobile phone, and slippers? If they live alone, should they call someone to accompany and stay with them? Older people recognize that they will become dependent upon strangers for their most basic needs—a frightening thought.

There is also a significant risk that an older person may get confused and angry in the acute hospital setting. It can be a threatening and very scary environment. If they get terrified and agitated, they will likely be restrained, physically or pharmacologically. After all, they are pulling out their IVs, tugging at their catheters, or taking off their oxygen mask. Restraints will make them even more confused, combative, and more agitated, resulting in even more restraints. This vicious circle can go around for a while. (See section below on surviving hospitalization.)

Fortunately, most of the time people feel sick, they do not need hospitalization. People should know that hospitals do not like to keep patients in their institution for long periods and don't rush to admit, unless the doctors themselves are worried and uncomfortable with caring for the individual at home. There are many issues of concern that influence the need to hospitalize: some medical, some social, some related to the environment and availability of services at home. Unfortunately for the older person, an aged person is far more likely to be hospitalized than a younger one. Their advanced age makes them frail, and serious illnesses may present in a more subtle manner in the aged, making the treating physicians more conservative in their recommendations and more worried about the outcome (although they may not openly show their fears).

Comment: Doctors who know the patient are far less likely to admit the patient or order extensive testing than doctors who have never seen the patient previously, so develop a relationship with your primary care doctor and keep the relationship current by regularly scheduled visits.

Managing an unexpected sudden illness

"I'm worried about my mother. She's behaving strangely today, and seems short of breath. She's not eating nor drinking, and is moaning. Should I bring her to the hospital?" Abrupt changes sometimes occur in an older person's status; often this is accompanied by an acute alteration in mental status (delirium), but sometimes there is a new onset of difficulty in breathing, pain, or stomach problems. The dramatic change in behavior or function usually triggers panic and fear in family members of some new calamity befalling the individual.

The brain, in older people, often is the most sensitive indicator of something being wrong, almost anywhere in the body; and a sudden change in mental status can be due to a heart attack, a gallbladder attack, dehydration, a stroke, a change in sodium or salt concentration in the blood, a change in the heart rhythm, or any new condition that alters the status quo in the body. A sudden change suggests there is a new player that has been added to the mix. The question is whether that player came from the outside, or a new event occurred on the inside.

The individual should be seen and examined by a physician or trained nurse practitioner (see below). It's best to start by looking for something new that has been added to the body, such as a new medication recently taken, or one recently removed from the medication list. An infection is a common new acquisition (and one that can be treated) that now adds a strain to the system—urinary and respiratory infections being the most common. Infections can be accompanied by greater dehydration and circulating toxic agents that affect many organs, including the brain. Often, a cause for the sudden change can be identified, and successfully managed.

Case example: An older woman, living alone, was found one morning undressed, confused, throwing food, and being quite agitated. She previously had a mild to moderate dementia, and was taking medicines for her dementia. She had been functioning mostly independently the day before, and this change in behavior was totally unexpected by her home attendant and family.

Comment: A search for the cause of this abrupt change in behavior revealed a new urinary infection, and after hydration and antibiotics, the older woman was back to her previous level of functioning.

Risks of surgery in the elderly

"The doctors want to operate on my eighty-five-year-old mother. Is this safe?" No surgery is perfectly safe, but surgery in eighty- and ninety-year-olds carries much greater risk than operating on a healthy twenty-year-old. But healthy twenty-year-olds rarely need surgery. There is much cause for concern with surgery in the elderly. Surgery is a trauma to the body as well as the psyche. Patients are generally worried, the family is worried, and doctors often are worried.

There are increased risks of infection during surgery and in the recovering post-op period, while the patient is at bed rest in the hospital and having IVs and urinary catheters. Particularly worrisome in the hospital setting is exposure to so many different germs that are difficult to treat because of their antibiotic resistance (such as MRSA).

There is an increased risk of developing blood clots in the deep veins of the legs (DVTs) with the prolonged bed rest that recovery usually entails. (This is why patients frequently are given special inflatable "booties" that squeeze the feet and lower legs, preventing stagnation and pooling of blood in leg veins, or are given anticoagulants to retard clotting.) In the elderly there may be delayed healing of wounds and wound infections. This is all in addition to any problems encountered with the surgery itself and with the condition that required the surgery.

To reduce the risk of complications, surgeons try to shorten the anesthesia time and limit the amount of tissue that needs cutting. They may try using minimally invasive and laparoscopic approaches if possible, and employ lasers and robotics during surgery. These techniques have led to shorter recovery periods and fewer postoperative complications, even in the very elderly.

With surgery there is a need for some form of anesthesia. General anesthesia is stressful for the aging brain. In older patients, anesthesia brings on more confusion and even delirium than seen in younger patients. Then there may be the IVs and catheters that are needed to deliver medications, monitors to assess basic functions, and surgical drains to remove any collecting inflammatory fluids from the surgery. These often cause more distress to and agitation in older patients with a mild dementia; these individuals don't understand why these tubes are even there, and may try to remove them. The stress of the surgery (or the stress of the underlying condition needing surgery) can stimulate the heart into irregular heart rhythms, chiefly atrial fibrillation (AF; see section below for details about AF).

The immobility and forced bed rest is more likely to result in skin damage to the older, more fragile skin of the elderly. Elderly patients heal more slowly and are more prone to postoperative wound infections because of the changes of aging in their functions of circulation, their skin, wound healing, and ability to fight germs. It usually takes much longer for the elderly to recover to the point they feel able to get out of bed and move around. But to reduce postoperative complications, staff will demand the patient be mobilized as soon as possible. Lastly, with more atherosclerosis and hardening of the arteries, circulation issues become more evident and worrisome. In eighty- and ninety-year-olds, the circulation to all organs in the body is already compromised to some extent. Adding inflammation (as with an inflamed gallbladder—cholecystitis—or intestinal diverticulum—diverticulitis) sometimes results in the organ's rupture or other severe complications.

Awareness of what can go wrong with and after surgery will help you understand better what the surgeon and anesthesiologist are saying, and what questions you should ask of them.

Surgeons often say that when operating on a healthy young person, they rarely have problems; but when they operate on an older individual, they always have complications, no matter how carefully they perform the surgery. If the older individual had had previous surgeries, the resultant internal scars will add to the difficulty of subsequent abdominal surgery. The problems originate from the individual, not the surgeon. And if the older individual also has diabetes, obesity, heart disease, hypertension, or requires medications for their heart, blood pressure, thyroid, adrenal function, etc., the complexity of their care and response to surgery becomes even more a worry.

The patient, or his proxy, must sign an *informed* consent for the proposed procedure before any surgery can be performed. The key word here is *informed*. The person obtaining the consent must inform the person consenting of all the possible complications that might occur. Any use of medical jargon or abbreviations should be avoided, or restated in language that is clear and understandable to everyone involved; any questions the patient may have should be answered to their satisfaction.

Hearing of all the things that can go wrong with the surgery can be very frightening. Remember that these are required warnings about events that occur very rarely, and that thousands of people are undergoing that same surgery daily without any serious difficulties.

Case example: A ninety-year-old woman has been having abdominal pains for three days. She has had blood in her urine, and a CT scan of her abdomen shows a kidney mass that was felt by the radiologist to represent a renal carcinoma. Surgery was recommended.

Comment: As with what I have been stressing in this book, the family needs to consider the value of surgery vs. the risk of surgery (with all the possible complications enumerated above). Will the surgery make her life better? If the pain she is having can be managed by nonsurgical means, the balance may favor nonsurgical, conservative therapy; but much depends upon her anticipated life expectancy and how her general health is faring. If her pain is persistent, and surgery seems the only practical means of giving her relief, the balance may tip in favor of surgery.

The impact and challenge of stroke

"I think my mother just had a stroke. Her speech is slurred and she looks confused." A stroke is a result of a portion of brain tissue that dies because it has lost its blood supply (a cerebral infarction). The amount of brain tissue affected is a function of the size of the artery occluded and the amount of brain tissue it supplied. A stroke is generally an acute event, and leaves the patient and family very frightened. Occasionally the stroke seems to evolve and get larger, due to the arterial blockage extending by virtue of the clot enlarging, more clots developing, or the circulation being reduced by pressure in the brain. If the stroke involves a large part of the brain, or involves critical areas that control breathing or other vital functions, the individual can rapidly lose consciousness and expire within a relatively short period. If vital functions are not affected, the person will have a variable deficit, and may live for many more years. Treatment and prevention of another stroke depend on what caused the stroke.

If seen by medical personnel in an emergency room within three hours of the event, neurovascular imaging can be done, and the affected artery or clot can be opened or dissolved respectively.

If blood supply can be reestablished before brain cell death occurs, the damage caused by the stroke can be aborted. Such action should be performed as soon as possible, as a delay of up to four and a half hours reduces the efficacy of such treatment. Such patients may subsequently be treated for life with medicines to reduce clotting and the risk of another stroke.

There are three kinds of strokes. The most common is a *thrombotic* stroke (wherein a clot develops in an artery that normally brings blood to the brain, thus depriving a portion of brain tissue of blood). An *embolic* stroke occurs when a clot, a cholesterol plaque, or any clump of solid material breaks into the bloodstream going to the brain and blocks an artery. A *hemorrhagic* stroke is one where an artery breaks or leaks, and blood escapes into the brain—in a manner analogous to a water pipe that leaks or bursts.

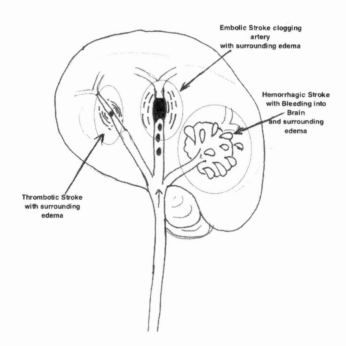

Fig. 1. Types of strokes: thrombotic, embolic, hemorrhagic

The cause for a thrombotic stroke is hardening and narrowing of arteries going to the brain (arteriosclerosis). A cholesterol plaque may rupture through the arterial inner lining, and rapidly produce a clot. As with arterial vascular disease elsewhere in the body, hypertension, smoking, diabetes, and high cholesterol are the most common reasons leading to the arterial narrowing. These also become the targets of therapy to reduce the risk of another stroke—ONE MUST REDUCE THESE RISKS. Many people take a small dose of aspirin (and sometimes a blood thinner) to reduce the risk of clotting.

Any part of the brain can be affected by the stroke, and the manifestations will vary depending upon what brain function is involved. What most people think of when they think about a stroke is one that affects the large artery that feeds the left part of the brain (the left carotid artery). The left side of the brain controls the right side of the body, and the afflicted person will lose speech, use of the right arm and leg, and have a drooping face. There can be problems with swallowing, facial weakness, and loss of vision on the right side. Strokes can be large and massive, or small and affect only limited functions (such as speech clarity or limb strength). Evolving strokes indicate that there is ongoing progressive loss of function. This suggests an enlarging clot that is affecting a greater zone of brain tissue.

Embolic strokes are seen mostly in individuals who suffer with atrial fibrillation. In atrial fibrillation, the atria are not beating effectively, but are merely "quivering." With stagnating blood in the atria, a blood clot may develop and break loose, free to travel along with the circulation. Since a large amount of blood goes to the brain, the risk of a stroke is substantial. The size of the clot will determine how far the clot can travel before it reaches an arterial branch who's narrowing diameter stops the clot. This determines the size of the stroke. Patients with atrial fibrillation are usually anticoagulated (taking a "blood thinner") for life to reduce blood clotting.

The brain occupies the space within the hard-sided skull. Anything added to this space, such as inflammatory cells, bleeding, or swelling (edema) caused by accumulation of fluid in response to the inflammation, takes up room and increases the pressure on the normal parts of the brain (very much like shoving more "stuff" into an already filled suitcase). The loss of brain function involves the immediate zone that loses blood supply (ground zero), but also a surrounding zone that receives less blood because of the pressure of inflammation. With time, the body can repair these marginal areas that received enough blood to keep brain cells alive (although not working very well). Other parts of the brain can sometimes be trained to learn new functions. The extent of healing may therefore take up to a year to finalize. There will always be some loss of function. Prompt rehabilitation is important. With therapy directed at "working" the affected functions, later problems (such as choking when swallowing, or developing frozen joints) can be avoided and maximal function during this healing process is allowed.

There is a phenomenon called a "transient ischemic attack, or a TIA—in this condition, there is complete resolution of the neurological findings within twenty-four hours. It is felt to be due to spasms of blood vessels, which only temporarily interrupt blood flow to the brain.

Migraine equivalents are also related to spasms of blood vessels and can produce diverse neurological alterations, which resolve with resolution of the spasm. These occur in individuals who generally have had a past history of migraine headaches, but may occur without any headache.

It should be noted that many older individuals commonly have had "silent" strokes or vascular occlusions that went unnoticed. When performing a sensitive MRI brain scan in a person older than seventy, it is almost certain that the radiologist will comment upon a "lacunar stroke" and microvascular disease. All older people have them. These have been produced by occlusions of small vessels, which went unnoticed at the time of their occurrence. Reading the report frightens the older patient, who then vigorously denies ever having had a stroke. The brain can take a lot of abuse and insult, and still keeps working.

Case example: An elderly man experienced a sudden loss of function on his right side. A special MRI of his brain demonstrated a new left-sided stroke. The time from the event till medical evaluation was twelve hours.

Comment: Survival will depend upon the individual's ability to breathe, swallow, or maintain other vital brain functions. Temporarily the individual may need a breathing tube and a feeding tube.

Feeling of weakness and generalized fatigue

"I feel very weak—I seem to have no energy, what's wrong with me?" Weakness is one of those ambiguous complaints that can signify any one of a number of underlying problems. It's analogous to saying, "My car doesn't go very well." There may be no immediate clue as to what system is responsible for this feeling, and where the doctor should begin the search to unravel the cause. Unfortunately, unlike modern cars, we are not made with a computer that can be interrogated to identify where the problem originates. As mentioned previously, aging is associated with a loss of energy, and "feeling weak" may be nothing more than the weakness of advanced age, but it would be a mistake to blame weakness on aging alone without a thorough work-up for other possible underlying conditions. This is particularly true if the weakness came on suddenly.

Weakness can be due to any major organ dysfunction, and is a common side effect of many medications. The work-up should include the exclusion of any adverse medication effect, a careful history of how and when the "weakness" developed; a good physical examination, and a standard battery of blood tests, which then may need additional follow-up testing with more specific tests. Muscle weakness or atrophy may be evident on physical examination. Watching the person walk or get up on the examining table can suggest a cause of the weakness. The initial battery of tests may indicate a failure of a specific organ, such as kidney, liver, or heart failure. Hormonal or endocrine abnormalities (such as thyroid disease, diabetes, adrenal, pituitary, sex hormone dysfunction), anemia, electrolyte abnormalities (such as abnormalities in acid levels, sodium, potassium, calcium, or iron) can be identified with these blood tests. Any significant abnormality in these areas, as well as many other deficiencies, can cause weakness.

Weakness and fatigue often are the reasons older people give as the reason they "need more rest." It is natural to rest when tired. However, as I remind my patients, rest never strengthens muscles or reverses weakness. It is exercise that improves stamina and strength and stimulates the body.

Weakness can also be a manifestation of depression. A cause for the weakness is usually identified without too much difficulty. The problem then becomes one of how to reverse the symptom. Patients frequently ask for an "energy pill," something that would give them strength and energy.

Comment: I sometimes recommend the "weak" individual go on a holiday to some romantic, exotic location. If they feel weak on such a vacation, it generally excludes depression as the cause, and gives the "weakness" a more objective measurement. This "test" is a lot more fun, and often much cheaper, than any other type of testing.

Feeling unsteady: balance, falling, and hip fractures

"I seem to be unsteady, and have to hold on to someone while walking. I'm worried about falling and about whether I have had a stroke." The complaint of imbalance should be a RED FLAG to the family and the doctor.

It is so very important in our lives to have good balance and protection against falling and fracturing our hips and shoulders. Independent living requires the person be able to get up and walk without the assistance of another person. Falls and hip fractures are arguably the most common cause for the end of independent living and the need for institutional living. Life expectancy after a fall and fracture is significantly reduced. Anything that can be done to prevent a fracture is well worth doing. Osteoporosis leads to weaker and more fragile bones. Fractures will occur if the force applied to the bone is strong enough to break it. Consider bone fractures that happen in healthy young athletes, or in anyone falling down stairs or being hit by a motor vehicle. If one falls enough times or with legs in the wrong position, a hip fracture will occur sooner or later. Osteoporosis and dizziness will be discussed below, but imbalance is a separate issue. Imbalance can be due to environmental factors (slippery floors, no bathroom mats or nonskid mats in the bathtub), or problems with the person's balance itself. It should be noted that the most common scenario seen with hip fractures is with older individuals who took sleeping pills, then had to go to the toilet during the night.

Balance problems can also be caused by medications that affect the brain. Sleeping pills, painkillers, and alcohol can all affect gait stability, reaction time, and balance, and thus can increase falling. Weakness (as described in the previous section) can cause imbalance and falling. Having previously fallen, fear of falling, loss of confidence in walking, and stiffness will increase the risk of future falling. When we learn to walk, ride a bicycle, ice skate, or ski, much of our success relates to a fluidity of movement, built on a confidence in our movement that is needed for these activities. When we become uncertain and afraid of falling, we become stiffer and more at risk of falling. In addition, with arthritis or pain in a joint or limb, this fluidity and movement of the joints may be compromised, and falls will be more common. Instability in gait and balance can be due to shifting the weight away from the painful joint before the shift in weight is complete.

Nerves (which are like wires transmitting electrical signals throughout our body) tell our brain where we are and what position our body is in. In various neurological disorders that are seen more frequently in the elderly, these messages are imperfect. With aging there can be back disease (as discussed below) and degenerative neurological disease causing neuropathy (neuro-pathology). Neuropathies can be associated with medications (particularly anti-cancer chemotherapy), Parkinson's disease, senile amyloid (caused by accumulation of proteinacious amyloid in the nerves), diabetes, thyroid disease, vitamin deficiencies, and some infectious diseases and malignancies. If the nerves are not working well, we lose the benefit of their normal function and signals.

Even without any significant nerve difficulties, *reaction time*—that interval of time from the moment the brain recognizes the need to make a movement till the time the movement begins—lengthens considerably with aging. The consequence of this normal aging process is that it takes longer for the older person to react with defensive movements in the event of a loss in balance. Many people, during the course of the year, slip, misstep, or stumble at some time or other, but, fortunately, catch themselves and don't fall. Older people will report that if they slip or stumble, they will fall; once they start going down, they will fall down.

There are devices to protect the hips when balance is poor. Hip protectors are Styrofoam sleeves that fit into pocketed undergarments that hug and protect the hips. In wearing them, the impact of a fall may not be transmitted to the hip directly in sufficient amount to cause a break. Corner protectors are soft cushions that can be placed over sharp corners of furniture, thus protecting against a rib fracture if a person stumbles and bangs their chest and ribs against the corner's point.

For the older person, the use of power-assist chairs can help patients stand and also ease their sitting so that they don't just "plop" into a chair, banging their heads against the wall and snapping their neck violently forward and back. Similarly, the use of lift-assist cushions, hospital beds, and side rails can be helpful to a handicapped person. Side rails on a bed may sound like a good way of preventing an individual from accidentally rolling off the bed, but they can be harmful, as people may feel restrained and may try to climb out of bed. Half rails, to help people lift and steady themselves as they get up from bed, are generally safer than full-length side rails. The use of physical (and even pharmacological) restraints has decreased in hospitals as we realize that they can be more harmful than helpful.

There are many types of assistive devices that are available and are covered by insurance if needed—too many to be listed here. But within any particular type of assistive device, there still are many, many choices to be made. It is important for someone in the family to review what kind of walker, or wheelchair, or power chair will be needed. The supply company can help, and will ask about the width of door frames, the type of flooring or carpeting, whether the device will be used indoors or out of doors, whether the older person can operate the device on their own (using the large outside rings attached to the wheels of the wheelchair), or will need to be pushed or manipulated by others. Other important questions that would need answering would be: "How long will the person be using the device during the day; will a wheelchair need a special cushion; is a lightweight collapsible device needed?" etc.

I recommend someone in the family go through the home with the eye of a "safety engineer." Is the bathroom safe? Should grab-bars be installed on any of the bathroom walls? Is lighting adequate? Is the furniture near the bed sturdy enough to support someone if they lose their balance and need to hold on? Should the chairs, toilet seat, couch be raised? (This would make getting up easier.) Are there hazards along the route going from the bedroom to the bathroom during the night, when the rooms are darkened? Should the kitchen dishes and utensils be moved to reduce the need for bending, or climbing on a step stool? But if climbing is necessary, using a sturdy step stool is infinitely better than standing on a chair. Avoiding a fall is much better than fixing a fracture.

Case example: Her housekeeper found an eighty-six-year-old woman lying on the floor of her bedroom when she came to work. The woman was soiled with urine, and had bruises and cuts on her face. Unable to get up alone, she had been lying on the floor for at least several hours. She claimed she slipped getting out of bed, while trying to go to the bathroom. An X-ray confirmed a hip fracture.

Comment: In addition to dealing with the damage caused by the fall, it is important to recognize whether the fall was the problem or the symptom of an underlying greater problem. The natural response to falling is to protect the face from trauma. When there is evidence of trauma to the face, there is a strong possibility that the individual had lost consciousness before the fall, having made no attempt to shield her face with her arms or hands. Lying on the floor for several hours can result in development of pressure ulcers (see below). Before the hip fracture can be repaired, she would need medical clearance, and evaluation of a pos-

sible cardiac or brain condition that caused her to "pass out" (see below under dizziness).

Feeling dizzy and having blackouts

"I am feeling very dizzy and lightheaded, am I having a stroke?" What is the significance of our older relative's complaint of always feeling dizzy? Dizziness is another common complaint in the elderly that leads to a great deal of testing and frustration on the part of the patient, their family, and the doctors caring for the patient. *Dizziness* is a very ambiguous term, and means different things to different people. In some people, it equates with light-headedness; in others, it is a premonition of an impending fainting spell; in still others, it is vertigo (where the room is spinning). Most often it is a benign condition associated with head positioning (benign positional vertigo, or BPV). Some people feel a sense of seasickness and describe it as dizzy. In still others, any abnormal sensation they feel in their brains is defined as dizziness. To help your doctor understand what you mean, try to use additional terms to describe your sensation—*dizziness* is too vague a term.

The causes for dizziness can be anything that interrupts the brain from getting what it needs for normal functioning (oxygen, nourishment in the way of blood glucose, and normal electrical stimulation in the way of brain waves). If a car engine does not get enough gas, air (as when the air filter is blocked), or if the engine timing is off, it will never run smoothly and efficiently. The same is true of the brain. The causes of dizziness can originate from the heart or arterial blood vessels bringing blood to the brain. Anything that reduces the blood supply to the brain can cause a variety of symptoms from light-headedness to blackouts. If the heart rhythm suddenly becomes erratic, pauses, or becomes too fast and irregular, it will pump blood less efficiently.

If the blood cannot get out of the heart (as when a heart valve is narrowed and does open adequately to allow enough blood to exit the heart), or if the blood pressure drops too rapidly or too much, the brain will not function normally.

A special form of dizziness is caused by a condition called orthostatic hypotension. This situation occurs when a person stands up from a lying or sitting position and feels dizzy or lightheaded. It is due to a drop in blood pressure that may occur with assuming an upright position—when gravity pulls the blood downward toward the legs, leaving less blood available for our brain. Each of us has, at one time or another (after being sick in bed for a day or two, after eating or drinking alcohol in excess), had this sensation. You feel dizzy or sense the room spinning when you try to stand, and immediately need to lie down again. In the elderly, there are a number of conditions that make this drop in blood pressure with standing (orthostatic) very common. Elderly people have slower nerve responses, with slower sensing and responding to the drop in pressure. Elderly people commonly take medications that lower blood pressure that can interfere with the body's ability to raise blood pressure rapidly, if it drops. With dehydration (a frequent finding in the elderly), the drop in blood pressure can be excessive and cause dizziness, falling, or blacking out (syncope). Many doctors recommend patients follow "the rule of ten" to manage this problem: from lying, to sitting, to standing, count to ten before going on to the next position. Wait till the head clears, then begin to walk.

Panic attacks and deep rapid breathing can bring on dizziness in any of us. Intense breathing reduces the carbon dioxide in the blood, lowers the acid level, and changes the concentration of free calcium. These effects can cause dizziness and blackouts. Breathing into a paper bag can be helpful, as the air in the bag will have a greater concentration of carbon dioxide.

Another form of dizziness, and even passing out, is called vasovagal. The cause of this form of syncope is an overstimulation of vagus nerve activity. Overstimulation of the vagus nerve slows the heart, drops blood pressure, and stimulates the intestines. This was the reason our parents always cautioned us about going out to play after a big meal. We were usually told that "all the blood was going to our stomach" and we would get sick if we tried to exercise. Vagal responses occur with overeating, overdrinking, upset stomach, irritation of the bowel, a large bowel movement, catheterization of the bladder, or any activity that irritates the gastrointestinal or urinary tracts. With a strong vagal response, the drop in blood pressure and slowing of the heart rate can be enough to reduce the blood flow to the brain, and dizziness or blacking out can occur. If the person with a vagal reaction tries to walk, they will siphon more blood away from their brain, sending it to their legs. Stricken individuals will feel dizzy, light-headed, sweaty, have decreased visual and hearing acuity, and can pass out if they don't quickly lie down. When lying down, gravity no longer acts to collect blood in the legs, and they don't need as great a blood pressure to circulate the blood to the brain; the individuals will feel better. As the irritation of the gastrointestinal track normalizes, the vagus nerve loses its overstimulation and the condition corrects itself. The trick in recognizing a vasovagal reaction is to measure the heart rate. With overstimulation of the vagus nerve, the heart rate will be very slow. With other conditions causing light-headedness or blackouts, the heart rate will be rapid.

In each of these conditions, the brain does not get its needed oxygen, glucose, or calcium, and the person is at risk of losing consciousness or just feeling dizzy. Sometimes turning the head or twisting the neck can compress the arteries that go to the brain and can cause dizziness. This can be seen when the person walks to the corner of the block and has to turn her head sideways, or look upward, to see oncoming traffic or the traffic light. Similarly, standing in the front of some elevators requires the neck to be tilted way back to see which floor the elevator indicator signals. If the blood vessels traveling up the back of the neck get pinched, the person can feel dizzy or pass out.

If the blood sugar drops too low, even with normal blood flow to the brain, the brain will not be getting enough glucose to fuel its metabolic need, and the person can lose consciousness or feel dizzy. This can happen easily in a diabetic person who takes her insulin, but does not eat or misses meals.

If the electrical activity of the brain becomes unstable (as with a seizure) the person may feel dizzy or pass out.

Sometimes the dizziness and fall is due to weakness caused by an infection. The infection can produce dehydration, loss of appetite, and generalized weakness. The dehydration increases the risk of orthostasis. When the person tries to stand and walk, they may feel unsteady, dizzy, and fall.

Dizziness can also be caused by problems in the inner ear, where the semicircular canals are located and where the vestibular nerve originates and carries information of how and where the body is moving and sends this information to the brain. Inner ear infections, labyrinthitis, Meniere's disease, and vestibular neuritis (inflammation of the vestibular nerve) all can cause dizziness.

The significance of the dizzy spells is great. Regardless of the cause, or what exactly is meant by *dizzy*, there is a risk of falling with its associated risk of fracture. The consequences can be severe, depending upon where the person is standing at the time of the dizziness (e.g., crossing a street, on an escalator, while cooking or carrying a hot object). Evaluation of the "dizzy-complaint" involves much questioning and testing, and may require referral to neurologists, ear/nose/throat (ENT) specialists, and cardiologists.

Case Example: While walking in the street, an elderly woman fell and fractured her hip. When brought to the hospital, the surgeons were called to repair the fracture. Internists were called to give "medical clearance." When asked why the person fell, the patient replied she tripped on uneven pavement. When asked how often she walked that same path over the uneven pavement, and why she had never tripped there before, she hesitated and had no answer.

Comment: People rarely accept personal responsibility for an accident (it is an admission of a failing), but rather try to excuse the accident by blaming something in the environment outside of themselves. This is a poor response, as it deflects attention away from searching for the real cause of the fall, and trying to prevent another one. Again, it is always best to discover whether the fall was the problem, or was the symptom of another underlying problem.

Suffering with insomnia and sleep disturbances

"I can't sleep without sleeping pills; they're no longer working well; why can't I just keep taking more of them every night?" The tragic death of Michael Jackson still rings in our ears, and should be a lesson to every one of all ages—TAKING SLEEPING PILLS IS NOT WITHOUT RISK! Why do so many older people complain of not being able to sleep, and rush to take sleeping pills? Sleep problems in an older person eventually affects many people in the family. It can be the focus of a person's very existence. The amount of sleep a person needs is not fixed in hours. If you feel rested and alert in the morning, you probably had enough sleep.

Causes for insomnia can be arthritic pain or discomfort while lying down, or a poor mattress on the bed that adds to the discomfort. The insomniac may have heart failure and feel short of breath when lying flat in a bed, but will sleep better in a recliner or resting semi-upright on a couch. But frequently the individual has been napping all day, and has actually already slept for many hours. Sleeping another eight hours at night is far more sleep time than the body requires. The problem is not one of not sleeping at night; it's of sleeping all day. Often, if a spouse has recently died, the remaining individual may have difficulty sleeping in the large bed alone. The natural pattern of life for all animals has been to be active during the day, to be stimulated by things in the environment, and at the end of the day, to feel tired and go to sleep.

After retirement, there is no set schedule placing demands on the older person's time; there may be no compelling need to get up early in the morning. The natural time clock in our brain (the hormonally driven circadian rhythm that gives us jet lag when we cross time zones, or awakens us at a given time, even without an alarm clock) often gets dysfunctional in the elderly. The natural rhythm of living is disturbed. Depression can lead to a lack of interest in the day's activities, and a desire to escape reality by sleep. If the person had always had a good sleeping pattern, the family should alert the physician of the change, as this may signal a more serious problem, for which the difficulty sleeping is only the presenting symptom.

There are sleep-therapists who help people get back to a normal pattern of sleep. They generally advise removing TVs from the bedroom, cooling the temperature of the nighttime bedroom, not lying down in bed till it's time for sleep, and getting up at a defined time. A sleep-diary is also very helpful. In a sleep-diary, a caregiver actually writes down and records the hours of sleep for the affected individual.

Some people take the oldest sleeping aid known to mankind—an alcoholic nightcap to help them sleep. Others take over-the-counter sleeping aids or ask their doctor for sleeping pills. But, as stated above, taking sleeping pills carries significant risk. These medicines affect brain function, sometimes even long after the person awakens (particularly in older people). Most sleep medicines are formulated to give the average consumer an eight-hour sleep. With aging, and slower metabolism, this eight-hour period can be stretched considerably, and some effects of the medicine can last long into the next day. If the individual has to get up at night to go to the bathroom, the risk of falls and hip fractures goes up considerably if the older person has taken a sleeping pill. No small wonder. It is dark, they waited till the last moment to make the decision to go to the bathroom, there may be obstacles (such as shoes or clothing) in the path to the bathroom, the brain is not fully awake, and now the sleeping pill makes the person even more groggy and unsteady. The over-the-counter medicines can also make a person more confused, groggy, with dry mouth, blurred vision, and constipated. These OTC medications contain diphenhydramine (Benadryl), a medication that should be avoided, if possible, in someone with mild dementia or memory loss (see *dementia* below). Statistics show it is this scenario: the nocturnal visit to the bathroom in someone who had taken a sleeping pill, which is most associated with hip fractures in the elderly. Furthermore, sleeping pills usually lose their efficacy in inducing prolonged sleep after several weeks of continued use. But after such regular and prolonged use, the person becomes dependent on them, and will not sleep if the medication is not taken. The body becomes adapted to the medicine effect, but now requires the sleeping medicine for even falling asleep. Intermittent, judicious use of sleeping medications, or varying the type of sleeping medicine taken, can delay the body's adaptation and dependence on any single drug, and can be helpful in some people.

If we ask the older person who is asking for sleeping pills how they would like the gift of more life (not life added when they are old, but life at their current age), they usually jump at the offer. If told that not sleeping gives them more functional time to live, they protest. Often it is not sleep that the person desires, but rather anesthesia ("Knock me out!"). During sleep there is no feeling of pain, discomfort, or reminder of the problems that may face the older individual when awake.

Another disturbing sleep problem is excessive sleeping during the day. This may present as narcolepsy, in its extreme form (in this condition, individuals fall asleep in the middle of activities). Sometimes this is due to not getting a restful sleep at night, as in obstructive sleep apnea (OSA). The problem in OSA is that the person literally stops breathing during the night due to obstruction of the airway, and the oxygen level falls (and carbon dioxide levels rise) as the breathing stops. It is the waking up that allows the person to breathe more deeply and raise their oxygen level. Drinking alcoholic beverages or taking sleeping pills at night in this condition is extremely dangerous, as oxygen levels can drop to very dangerous levels without the person awakening. Seizures caused by too low an oxygen level can occur; there is a greater risk of heart attacks, dangerous heart rhythm disturbances, and hypertension caused by increased adrenalin secretion. By not sleeping at night, the affected person sleeps most of the day. Various nasal and oral appliances have had some success in reducing OSA, but patients usually require CPAP (continuous positive airway pressure), or surgery to correct the problem.

Experiencing nocturnal cramps in the legs, or having uncontrolled movements of one's legs (restless leg syndrome) are two other treatable conditions that might prevent effective sleep.

Dry eyes caused by dry air in the house (see below), can also cause excessive daytime sleepiness. The irritated dry eyes feel better when the eyelids are closed; closed eyelids invite sleep; it decreases visual stimulation, is restful, and the person can doze off. The use of humidifiers, earplugs, eyeshades, or soothing music can often help with sleep.

The body generally demands its sleep time. If a normal younger person is deprived of sleep, they eventually fall asleep in the middle of whatever they are doing. This can be a particular problem if they are driving a car. Sleep problems are a big problem and deserve serious attention. It requires a lot more consideration and thought then just prescribing or taking sleeping pills.

Case Example: Family members complain that they cannot retain a home health aid for their mother, who never sleeps, and prevents the attendant from sleeping as well. The attendant is threatening to leave, and the children are panicked about how to manage the parent's insomnia. They are requesting, even demanding sleeping pills be given their parent.

Comment: The children of this older person may not understand the risks associated with sleeping pills, and the reason their parent can't sleep. Rather than asking for a specific therapy, the children should outline the problem, and let the doctor make the decision of how best to handle the parent's insomnia.

Feeling numbness and tingling in the fingers

"Why do I have this numbness or tingling in the fingers of my hand when I wake up in the morning? Do I have multiple sclerosis?" Numbness is a common feeling that many older people have, and often then worry about whether it is a sign of a stroke, or an early manifestation of multiple sclerosis. What produces these symptoms is an irritation of the nerves that originate in the hand. As the nerves exit the hand on the way to the brain, they must traverse a narrow channel in the wrist called a carpal tunnel (the wrist bones are called carpal bones). There are a lot of moving bones in our wrist, and we have narrow wrists. Through this carpal tunnel pass nerves, tendons, and blood vessels—a lot of stuff. If there is some irritation or swelling that causes pressure on the tunnel, the nerves can get pinched. Depending upon how the person's wrist is positioned at night, there may be more compression of the tunnel and more symptoms in the morning.

After traversing the wrist, on the way to the brain, the nerves meet the next hurdle at the elbow, where a large nerve runs very close to the elbow joint. This is a less defined tunnel, but is sometimes called an ulna tunnel. If we bang our elbow, we feel the tingling and numbness that we attribute to "hitting our funny bone." The ulna nerve, one of the nerves coming from our hand, runs very close to the surface of the skin and next to an elbow bone; it easily can be irritated at this location by banging our elbows or resting our arms on a car window frame.

After passing by the elbow, the nerves go through our armpits (the axilla), where they rarely get compressed, but then the nerves must enter the spinal cord, going through an opening in the vertebra of our necks. Here is the second most common cause of the numbness and tingling of the fingers. Arthritis in our necks is almost always present as we get older, and the way we twist our necks on the pillow can cause irritation to the nerves.

As a point of information, numbness and tingling in the toes is also common and can be caused by wearing too constrictive shoes or pinching the nerves going from the foot to the brain (as with arthritis in our back).

Neurologists can often help identify the site of the nerve irritation, but may want X-rays of the neck and nerve-conduction tests to see where the nerve is irritated in more complex cases. Treatments may include surgery to open the carpal tunnel, wearing wrist splints at night, or cervical pillows (if the point of irritation is in the neck).

Aside from nerves becoming entrapped or pinched, the tendons in our fingers may get trapped as they traverse the two closer joints of the finger. This trapping produces a "trigger finger." The constant opening and closing of the fist requires these tendons slide back and forth through the sheaths surrounding the small joints of our hand, as our fingers open and close. If the tendons become irritated and swollen, they will "rub" as they pass through the joint sheath, and a swelling or nodule will develop at the site of irritation. Since the muscles involved in closing our fingers while making a fist are much stronger than those involved in opening our hands, we have little problem with closing our grip, but lack the strength to open or extend the involved finger. We may need to use our other hand to "snap open" the involved digit. This is called a trigger finger. It can be treated by reducing the irritation to the tendon by resting the finger with a splint, injection of cortisone into the tendon sheath, or by means of a surgical opening of the constriction.

Case Example: An older woman has been dropping objects from her right hand, feels weakness in the hand, and had been reluctant to complain about this to her family.

Comment: In time, carpal tunnel syndrome can become so severe that there is loss of nerve impulse transmission to the muscles of the hand, and atrophy of the large thumb muscle can be seen, with weakness of the grip. These cases require surgical intervention, which is a relatively simple and safe procedure that normally does not require an overnight stay in the hospital.

Annoying tremors and shaking in your hands

"What does it mean when my hands tremble?" Many elderly people develop tremors in their hands. They usually worry that they are developing Parkinson's disease when this happens. Aside from causing worry, the tremors can have an impact on the person's ability to button clothing, drink soup from a spoon, or write with a pen. What causes shaking, and what can be done?

Parkinson's disease is associated with a tremor at rest, while most of the tremors that occur in the elderly happen when they try to do things, and is caused by an "essential" tremor. This type of tremor is also variably called an action tremor, a familial tremor, or a senile tremor. There may be a head bob. The essential tremor, although developing later in life, is usually inherited, and can be aggravated by caffeine, as well as by certain medications (those containing adrenalin, ephedrine, amphetamines, or aminophylline). These drugs are mostly given to treat asthma, allergies, or "stuffiness" and runny noses. Too much thyroid hormone activity (as can occur with disease as well as taking too much replacement thyroid hormone) will cause a tremor. Increased anxiety and stress can cause an action tremor. In each of these cases, it seems to be due to too great a stimulant effect of adrenalin-like action on the nerves and muscles. It can be very bothersome to the individual, and it may be very embarrassing to them. If it bothers the person, it warrants therapy, and there are different medical treatments available. In severe cases of tremor, implanted wires in specific parts of the brain can often stop the shaking when the individual activates the electrodes.

Patients with Parkinson's disease frequently have a resting tremor that decreases when they try to do something. The main feature of Parkinson's disease, however, is rigidity, not tremor. Other types of tremors are seen with alcohol withdrawal (DTs, or delirium tremens), weakness and muscle fatigue, and some various other less-common brain and neurological disorders.

Case Example: An older man has had increased shaking and tremors in his hands when he tries to do something. His handwriting has become a scratchy scrawl and is barely legible. He can no longer write checks or notes. His children have bought him a computer and printer for him to use. He doesn't have the dexterity to use a cell phone, and has problems using utensils.

Comment: We need dexterity in our hands for so many of the common tasks we take for granted. A severe tremor can make us disabled and in need of help with almost anything we do. The patient and his family have to decide how aggressively they want to attack the problem.

Having a degenerative disease

"Is there any cure or anything that can be done for my arthritis?" Degenerative diseases, by their very nature and definition, are chronic, progressive, and debilitating. However, depending upon the underlying condition, there are a lot of things that can be done to reduce pain and improve function. There are a variety of degenerative disorders, whose cause is not now well understood, but where therapies exist to reduce the severity and symptoms of the disease. Neurologically these include Parkinson's disease, multiple sclerosis, Alzheimer's disease, and progressive degenerative brain palsies. Some of these disorders seem to have inherited predispositions. These degenerative diseases are all currently incurable disorders, which occur mostly in the elderly and usually cause significant disability and suffering (to the affected individual as well as to the family). We have some understanding of these conditions, and some treatments do exist that can help the affected person live a more normal life. Research continues to search for an inciting cause for these disorders. The infectious agents being considered are viruses and prions (small little pieces of nucleic acid that appear to be responsible for such disorders as mad cow disease). Other degenerative diseases involve our joints and bones, such as osteoarthritis, rheumatoid arthritis, scleroderma, and Crohn's disease. Here too, there are treatments, but no cures.

Infectious causes for these diseases are still being studied, but in the progression of these disorders there may be an imbalance between injury and repair functions. There may be an element of one's own defenses trying to stop the illness by a vigorous immune response, but causing more damage in the process (an autoimmune component). Many current therapies are aimed at reducing the immune and inflammatory responses. Hope lies with the newly advancing field of regulation of inflammatory conditions, and stem-cell research, which may provide cells which are "younger" and have not yet lost any of their "natural" functions.

Comment: The primary doctor, in concert with a neurologist or a rheumatologist, usually manages these degenerative disorders. Patients should not expect cures, but rather a way of ameliorating the problems.

Fear of dementia

"I don't know why my children brought me here, I feel well." People who are developing dementia usually try to hide their difficulty, and deny fiercely any problem they might have, or reference to memory loss. Dementia is probably the single most feared condition of people as they ponder aging. As mentioned earlier, a mild cognitive impairment (MCI) can be detected in many elderly persons. It may not progress any further in some individuals; but in others, it progresses to a dementia. MCIs are now being separated by whether there is a problem with memory alone (anamnestic MCI), single-function, or multiple-function MCI. There seems to be a difference in risk of evolving into a dementia between these various subtypes of MCI.

Dementia is feared as much, if not more, by family members as by the affected individual. As mentioned previously, the goal of living should not be to die with the best memory. As with many other disorders, if the individual is comfortable and enjoying many aspects of life, what does the diagnosis of "dementia" really signify? There are many diagnoses that carry even worse prognoses. Would it have been better if there were a diagnosis that the heart wasn't working well, or there was a failure in the function of the lungs, the kidneys, or the liver? Why should we single out dementia as the most feared diagnosis? Each of these disorders can progress to a point where the affected individual is severely handicapped and requires assistance with normal daily activities; none are good diagnoses. With dementia, however, the affected individual may not suffer the effects of the incapacity as much as with the other conditions. But it is a different type of burden to the individual with dementia and his family. Some degree of memory loss appears to be inevitable in the extremely old. It may be because of the image we have of what a demented person may become, and how they need care. We are uncomfortable with seeing an older family member, whom we had loved and admired, with a disorder that affects their cognition. Would we have accepted their sudden death with less distress?

As with many other organs that have lost much of their "reserve," the older brain is more sensitive to the effects of agents that may potentially affect its function. The older brain is at risk for any sudden decrease in circulation caused by changes in blood pressure, or arterial narrowing (which affect brain function by reducing blood flow), and changes in blood sugar or hydration (which can occur in diabetics or persons at risk for dehydration). In addition, many agents and medications can have significant impact on the function of the brain in older people. These include anesthetics, stimulants, muscle relaxants, antihistamines, alcohol, sleeping pills, antidepressants, antispasmodics (as used in relaxation of the bladder or bowel), as well as in many other different prescribed medicines (too many to list here). Special attention to potential changes in brain function must be taken when beginning any new medication, especially any of the above types of medicines. If brain function seems to be affected, the doctor should be notified, and stopping the offending medication should be seriously considered.

I should emphasize that these medications and changes in body functions (physiological changes) do not cause dementia. However, they can affect brain function to various degrees, and thus spark concern in the affected individual that a dementia is beginning.

Relatively early in a dementia, the person will try to hide his or her difficulty and will try to avoid new and frightening environments. They will avoid challenge. They do better in an environment in which they feel safe and secure—unthreatened. This is expressed by not wanting to go out and socialize. It also means they prefer not interacting with strangers, and keeping their environment as unchanging as possible.

People who are aware or concerned with memory loss need to be followed regularly, and tested periodically to see if their brain function is deteriorating, and whether they need treatment. Medical testing includes study of thyroid abnormalities, vitamin deficiencies, circulation problems, infections of the brain. They should have some brain-imaging study, such as an MRI. There are batteries of tests that look for depression, and examine different aspects of brain function (e.g., executive function, abstract thinking, recognition).

There are many types of dementia, which vary slightly, one from another, but seem to progress to a common state where the person affected is no longer able to function. The term *dementia* is distinct from the term *delirium*. The latter term refers to an acute process where the person's brain is suddenly not functioning well. Delirium is usually reversible and has an identifiable cause. Dementia is a chronic process, progressing slowly over a long period of time, and eventually involving all aspects of brain function. Dementia is much more than memory loss. It involves loss of judgment, calculations, orientation, and eventually all higher brain functions. Alzheimer's disease and/or vascular disease, affecting the blood supply to the brain, are the most common dementias seen in the elderly. A fronto-temporal form of dementia (FTD) has a somewhat different pattern of presentation and progression. This disorder (which had previously been called Pick's disease) generally presents at a younger age than the dementia of Alzheimer's disease. Language and behavioral abnormalities are the hallmark of FTD. Sometimes there are abnormal movements of the limbs. The progression of the disease seems to be more aggressive than other dementias, with a four-to-six-year life expectancy with this dementia (Alzheimer's disease patients generally have a six-to-ten-year life expectancy). Parkinson's disease may progress to a dementia that mimics the other dementias. A possible variant of Parkinson's dementia is a Lewy body dementia. Lewy bodies are found by microscopic examination of the brain, where brain cells have abnormal staining material inside the cell. Parkinson's disease patients also have these Lewy bodies in their brain cells. Hydrocephalus in the elderly (normal pressure hydrocephalus, or NPH) occurs when the drainage of spinal fluid cannot keep pace with the production of fluid. This condition produces problems with balance and gait, urinary control, as well as memory and word-finding difficulties early in its course. Patients fall frequently, often backward. They have a distinctive gait, with small uncertain steps. It is a condition not to be missed, as there is specific treatment for this condition (insertion of a shunt to drain the fluid). Many types of degenerative neurological disease seem capable of producing a dementia. Treatments are generally the same, and may help the manifestations of the disorder, but there are no cures available at present.

The assessment of dementia is usually done with mental status examinations, and patients scored by how well they perform. However, conditions such as anxiety, language difficulty, hearing, mental concentration, and a variety of ancillary medical conditions at the time of examination can all affect the results. An assessment of dementia that I find very informative is how the individual spends their free time and how they live. If they previously had enjoyed reading, can they still read novels or books with story lines or complicated information? In reading a novel, the reader must keep track of the characters and plot from one chapter to the next. If they had previously enjoyed movies, can they keep the plot and characters in memory during the 90–120 minutes most movies require? As dementia progresses, watching TV becomes limited to variety shows, sports, or game shows, which make no demands on concentration or remembering a story line.

Families of patients with dementia almost always worry about the risk of developing dementia in themself or in their children. There are genetic predispositions to developing dementia, and commercial tests exist for testing for some of these (as, for example, the apoE4 status, which was widely publicized in dementias developing in sports figures with head trauma). Examination of spinal fluid for Tau proteins is another diagnostic test that has been highlighted in the media. The FDA has recently approved the use of an antibody to detect abnormal amyloid accumulation in the brain (another manifestation of Alzheimer's disease). The hesitation in routine testing for these conditions lies in the lack of being able to do anything about the results, and how finding a "positive" test result will only produce significant anxiety and terror.

Much research is being done on dementia. Although we still don't understand the cause of Alzheimer's disease, we recognize certain pathological changes that occur in the brains of affected individuals, and can trace the deterioration to loss of chemical transmitters in specific parts of the brain. Nerve circuitry is different from electrical circuitry. Wires must touch one another to carry electrical current. Nerves transmit "current" by chemical transmitters that carry the impulse across the spaces between nerves. Of note is that these chemical transmitters can be affected by many commonly used medications (prescription and over-the-counter). Medicines that treat allergies, bladder irritability, and over-the-counter sleep medicines can make the dementia worse. At this time, there are only several approved medicines to treat Alzheimer's disease, none of which cure the disorder. They may, however, slow the progression of the dementia in some of the treated patients, and keep the person functioning more independently for a considerable time.

Management of vascular dementias focuses on keeping the individual's blood pressure, cholesterol, and circulation optimal.

Aside from treating the dementia, it is important to manage the behavioral problems that often are seen in dementia. The person with an early dementia may become agitated, strike out at family and those closest to them, and blame others for "things happening" in their lives. They may wander, have hallucinations, become frightened, and might not recognize friends and family. Many "sun down," defined as a change in their behavior at the end of the day, when the sun sets. Usually, it is expressed as greater confusion or agitation in the evening. This condition is seen most often in mild to moderate dementing disorders, and may respond to anti-dementia therapy. In mild to moderate dementia, people may become paranoid and suspicious of the motives of members in their family. They may cause havoc in the lives of their extended family. Families generally realize it is the disease that is behaving this way, and their loved one is unable to control the disease. Getting angry with the demented person, or becoming more upset and fighting back, can only worsen the affected person's behavioral problems. A rational discussion, trying to convince the affected individual that there is a problem in his or her brain, will never work, but can only increase stress. Treatment of these behavioral changes is frequently more important than treating the memory and judgment problems of dementia. Music can be tried as an adjunctive therapy to calm the affected person in a safe way (see below).

Case example: An older man was brought to the doctor's office. His children were disturbed by his memory loss and change in his behavior. They used a ruse to bring him in, claiming he was coming along to accompany an adult child who had the doctor's appointment. When the doctor started asking the patient his problems, the older man became angry and upset with his children and tried to leave.

Comment: This scenario is quite common. Using such a ruse to get the older person to the doctor can lead to more problems, when the older person feels their children are part of a conspiracy to hurt them. Fortunately they may not remember this for any long period, and may calm down if they feel the doctor is not being too threatening. Sometimes children appeal to their parent's sense of responsibility and get the individual to the doctor with the plea of "Do this for me—I am so worried about you that I can't sleep or function." Another way to get the demented individual into "the system" is to wait for something to "crash"—which in time will happen. Police or emergency personnel then take the demented person to a hospital emergency room, which is even more threatening to the older person than the doctor's office.

The cloud of depression

"I worry that I'm losing my memory, and have trouble sleeping." Depression is a common cause of memory loss in the older individual (pseudo-dementia). In the condition of pseudo-dementia, the individual usually complains about their loss of memory. In true dementia, they usually attempt to hide their memory loss (see above).

If one lives long enough, many individuals who are important in an individual's life will be gone: their spouse, siblings, friends, et al. They will ruminate about their own mortality, and can no longer hide from reality. If one takes the time to think about it, one can easily develop long lists of reasons for an aging person to become depressed. The signs of depression may be that of not eating (or eating too much), increased alcohol intake, poor grooming, isolation from friends and family, sloppy appearance, not wanting to get up in the morning, and lack of general interest in anything. They may complain of just "being tired all time" and wanting to lie in bed.

External as well as internal stress may increase depression. Depression is the one condition that most deprives the individual of their most valuable attribute—their ability to enjoy life. It will affect the entire family, one way or another. It therefore should be a top priority requiring attention; it is usually treatable, or often resolves by itself with time. This point needs emphasizing; without specific therapy, most depressive states in the elderly resolve in time by themselves.

In every age, there are stresses and reasons to be depressed and anxious, as well as opportunities for pleasure and enjoying life. Much has to do with the individual's basic makeup and outlook. Many people were depressed when they were younger and their depression merely continues. They are chronically depressed individuals. Families frequently mention their concerns about depression in their elderly relative, and inquire about medications to treat the depression.

A disturbing statistic is that suicide is a significant cause for mortality in the aged. Sometimes this occurs in the midst of acute grief caused by a spouse's death, sometimes due to the discovery of having a feared disease, sometimes simply because of loneliness and depression.

There are many ways to manage the loneliness and depression of the aged. Socialization is an important issue. Humans are social creatures, and if the spouse is gone, loneliness is a natural consequence. Getting involved in programs at senior centers or places of worship, taking courses at museums or local schools, beginning projects, learning new skills, traveling, talking to clergy and friends can all be helpful. Psychologists, psychiatrists, social workers, and good friends can play a helpful role. As a last resort, there are many medicines that can help the depression. It is important to differentiate grief from depression. Grief is a natural and normal response to tragedy. When it drags on and interferes with a person's ability to function, it is depression, becomes a significant medical issue, and needs treatment.

I am a firm exponent of trying music to assist in combating both depression and agitated behavior in demented patients. Music awareness, memory for music, and rhythm are localized in the *right* side of the brain (it is the left side of the brain that is the dominant hemisphere in right-handed individuals, controlling speech and most intellectual functions). Music can be used to calm agitated individuals and modify mood. It is safe, with no potential for abuse or adverse reaction. Listening to old songs that were enjoyed years ago may trigger more pleasant memories. Medications for depression may also be needed. But, unlike music, medications have potential side effects. If the person has a long history of depression and psychiatric disturbances, the depression may be more severe, and may require hospitalization and even shock therapy.

Case Example: An older parent seems to be eating less, becomes sloppy in appearance, and spends as much time in bed as possible. He or she is losing weight, and is getting weaker. The parent never wants to leave the home, and seems to have no interest in life. Even the visits of the grandchildren don't seem to be effective in getting him or her "up." The family is inquiring about the parent taking antidepressants.

Comment: There are many causes for the parent to be behaving as mentioned. A good medical evaluation should be the way to start, excluding dementia, neurologic disease, hormone deficiencies, or chronic infections as the cause. Antidepressants may certainly have a role in helping this person, but depression should not be the sole immediate diagnosis.

Significance of heart failure and palpitations

"I was told I have heart failure; what does this mean?" The term *heart failure* sounds very ominous. It suggests to the average person that the heart has worn itself out and is about to stop or has become no longer able to beat adequately. Actually, heart failure really means that the tissues of the body are not getting enough blood and oxygen, regardless of how well the heart is beating. Anemia can be a cause of heart failure. Heart failure is a relative term, can usually be treated and often reversed, may represent only an immediate condition, and may not as bad as it sounds. The degree of heart failure can be assessed by blood tests and echocardiograms.

So why do hearts develop heart failure? Usually this is due to the heart muscle being exhausted and not working well. Despite being filled with blood, the heart gets its nourishment from blood coming in through the coronary arteries. These arteries, like arteries elsewhere in the body, become more rigid, calcified, and narrow with plaque as we age. If the supply of blood through the coronary arteries becomes inadequate, the person will develop chest pain (angina pectoris) with exercise, which will subside with rest. The individual will be diagnosed with atherosclerotic heart disease. The harder the heart works (a function of heart rate and blood pressure), the more oxygen and fuel it will need; if there is not enough blood supply, pain develops. If the blood flow stops, the person has a heart attack, and some of the heart muscle dies (an *infarction*). The remaining muscle of the heart must pick up the loss. Problems with the functioning of the heart muscle itself are called cardiomyopathies (pathology in the muscle of the heart). Cardiomyopathies are often inherited.

Chronically high blood pressure stresses the heart, which has to pump against this pressure. With time, the muscle of the heart fatigues and can no longer meet the stress, and heart failure develops with hypertensive cardiomyopathy. Heart muscle actually remodels itself with changes in stress to the heart.

With aging, the muscle of the heart also becomes more rigid. The increased rigidity of the heart chambers restricts their relaxation and filling. This in turn results in less blood being pumped out with each beat. If the heart muscle "stretches" too much, or does not have enough blood nourishment, the force of contraction will diminish, and heart failure will develop. Some nutritional deficiencies and some infections in the heart can damage the heart muscle and lead to heart failure.

Heart valves also become more rigid with age. Valves may develop calcifications, may not close completely (leaking valves), or may not be able to open completely (tight, or stenotic, valves). Many elderly patients are shocked when they hear they have a "heart murmur" (noises of blood flow in the heart). They assumed their heart valves would remain pliable for their entire life and never leak. Like a slowly dripping faucet, a small leak may have no meaningful significance. Severe leaking or stenotic valves are a different story, and decrease significantly the efficiency of the heart function. Valves can be fixed or replaced if their malfunction is making a significant impact on heart-pumping efficiency. The individual will know if they are in significant heart failure, as they will become short of breath with minimal exertion. Although, as already mentioned, the term *heart failure* generally causes the individual to panic, heart function can improve with medications, or by relief of the conditions that were responsible for its development. It can change considerably, as measured by how well it empties the blood in its chambers when seen by echocardiogram. In general, it is much better to listen to how your body is working than to worry about the terminology or the natural aging of the heart.

In addition to problems with the muscle of the heart, aging can cause problems with the electrical activity of the heart. Most people over the age of sixty have "extra" beats. Generally these are benign and produce no symptoms. When these extra beats occur frequently, or in protracted runs of rapid beats, the efficiency of the heart pumping can drop significantly. Each heartbeat ejects a defined and measurable amount of blood. This blood exits as a rapid surge into an already blood filled aorta. The added volume distends the aorta, and increases the pressure of blood in the artery. The surge passes through the arterial system as a wave, and is felt as the pulse. After the wave passes, the pressure in the artery falls back to the "resting" pressure, before the wave came. These two pressures are termed the systolic and diastolic blood pressure respectively. When the heart is beating irregularly, the volume of blood ejected varies between beats, being dependent, among other things, upon how much filling time the heart experienced between beats. A longer filling time means more blood to be ejected, and a shorter filling time, less blood. In AF, with the most irregular rhythm, there will be great variations in the amount of blood ejected between beats, and therefore great variations in the measured blood pressure. (The significance of this is that people in atrial fibrillation should not focus on the actual numbers measured, but should discuss the number with their doctor). The irregular rate of AF may be too fast for satisfactory pressure and volume output, and the afflicted individual will feel lightheaded and short of breath. Slowing the *rate* of AF is more important than controlling the *rhythm*. Stagnating blood in the fibrillating atria may clot (as described on p. 47). To lower the risk of developing an embolic stroke, people with AF are usually anticoagulated. The causes for the onset of AF are several, and should be investigated. Some causes are treatable and reversible.

Since the elderly heart functions better when in a normal rhythm, doctors will sometimes try to "cardiovert" the heart back into a normal rhythm by an electrical shock or with medicines, and use medicines to stabilize the newly recovered normal rhythm. Such conversion of the irregular heart rate to a regular one requires the patient be shown not to already have a clot in her atrium. If a clot were to be found, the person would need anticoagulation for several months before an attempt at cardioversion. If a clot were to be present, the sudden beating of the atria allows a clot to be "pumped out" into the general circulation.

Case example: An older man has developed more shortness of breath (dyspnea) when walking or climbing stairs. He can no longer walk more than half a block before having to stop and rest. His doctor did testing, and diagnosed him with congestive heart failure.

Comment: With diuretics, medicines to reduce his blood pressure and heart rate, the patient lost eight pounds of excess fluid and was able to return to his previous level of activity without having to stop. An easy way to keep on top of heart failure is to weigh oneself daily. Absolute weight is unimportant—change in weight is. Water or fluid retention or loss can change the weight significantly from one day to the next; gain or loss of flesh rarely changes the weight more than one lb./day. A sudden large change in weight signifies fluid retention or loss, and the doctor should be notified.

The predictive value in screening for cardiovascular disease

"I read that there are a lot of sophisticated tests that can look at my circulation and can tell if I'm going to develop an heart attack"; "I would like to get these newer vascular studies to see how good my arteries are functioning, and would also like to have total body MRIs to look for any cancers." As with cancers (discussed in a later section), many people worry throughout their lives about "hidden diseases" and want to know if they are at risk of having a stroke or heart attack. (Note: if you are alive, you are at risk.) This anxiety is reinforced by unexpected deaths and disease they observe in their social contacts or are publicized in the news media.

One should realize that the more sensitive and sophisticated testing we do, the more small irregularities we must find. We are not all alike, and the more carefully we look, the more little differences between each other we will find; these usually have no functional significance. "How long have these 'irregularities' been there, and what is their significance?" We do have newer sophisticated vascular tests, and can look into the heart and arteries to examine the circulation and heart valves—but to what end, and for what benefit? With aging, we cannot expect to have the same arteries we had as when we were younger. Our heart valves and heart muscle will be stiffer, and we can have murmurs or bruits (noise of blood flow in arteries). We all will develop heart rhythm irregularities. So what! If we're not bothered by the problems, why look? New, sophisticated tests will always make the news as breakthroughs in diagnostic methodology. People frequently run to their doctors to ask for these newer tests. The problem is that these new tests have not yet been tested long enough to understand what their results indicate. There is no point of reference. It is only when, with time and experience, these tests have been used and evaluated can their results be put into perspective and their usefulness understood.

Doing routine screening will usually find some irregularity. It then cannot be ignored (otherwise, why did we do the test?). This will lead to further testing, more consultations, and more anxiety in the individual and their family. The general wisdom is to do more advance testing, not as a fishing expedition, but only when symptoms, or physical findings initiate a concern in the doctor (unless this is part of a research study).

Stress tests are an exception. Although there is a risk in stressing an older person's heart, it is safer and better to do this in a controlled and more protected environment, like a cardiac stress lab, than in a gym or on a ski slope. There are pharmacological stress tests available for individuals who cannot walk on a treadmill or ride on a bicycle. The predictive value of a stress test can be increased by coupling it with studies of how the heart circulation performs with a radionuclide test (a radioactive measure of blood flow to the heart muscle), or with echocardiography (which looks at muscle and valve function) with exercise. How often should we do these expensive tests? At present the indications are to evaluate the heart circulation before a person undergoes vascular surgery or any extensive surgery that can put the heart into stress, a strenuous newly planned exercise program, or if the symptoms suggest there may be a new problem with the circulation to the heart.

Still, we hear of people we know who, shortly after having gotten a clean bill of health, having undergone a medical examination, cardiac stress testing, and possibly even a vascular study of the arteries with catheterization and coronary artery X-rays (coronary angiograms), sustain a sudden heart attack. (A heart attack means that heart muscle tissue has died because of interruption of the blood flow to the tissue.) Having a heart attack after such medical reassurance is very disturbing to the patient, to those who hear about it, and to the doctor. The truth is that an unanticipated occlusion of an artery to the heart can happen suddenly and dramatically when the lining that covers an arterial cholesterol plaque suddenly tears. This is a new event that even the prior medical evaluation would not have detected. Screening test results bring no guarantees—only likely risk.

At this time in our medical sophistication, there is no 100 percent accurate way to predict a heart attack or to be certain there will be no heart attack. Although most heart attacks are associated with symptoms of chest pain, sweating, weakness, nausea, or passing out, in the elderly population, many have had heart attacks that neither they, nor anyone around them (including their doctors), had realized. After a routine EKG it can be a great surprise when the evidence of a past heart attack is indicated. Obviously they survived the injury without even the slightest awareness of the event nor any complaint about the consequence. (This is another important point about aging: serious illnesses may not have the same dramatic presentation and expression as one might expect in younger people.) If, however, the heart attack is recognized, early intervention with dissolving the clot, or opening the clogged artery before there is significant muscle death, can save heart tissue.

Case example: An older man has been having dizzy spells and doesn't feel well. On examination he was felt to have a problem with the circulation in his carotid artery carrying blood to his brain. A vascular study showed the artery to be 90 percent occluded, and the vascular surgeons wanted to operate on the artery as soon as possible. A stress test was done during the medical evaluation for clearance, and the result showed the patient had significant coronary artery disease. (It should not be surprising that more than one artery in an individual can have significant narrowing—after all, all the arteries have been subjected to the same levels of cholesterol, smoking, and stress.) The man underwent cardiac catheterization and angiography, revealing severe narrowing of one of his major coronary arteries. He had a stent (an expandable mesh tube) inserted into the coronary artery to keep it open. Surgery on the carotid artery to the neck was postponed till he was shown to be stable, and he underwent the carotid surgery several weeks later.

Comment: Although the patient had no symptoms of hardening of the arteries to his heart, it was necessary to evaluate his heart function prior to vascular surgery on his carotid artery. If this had not been done, the patient would probably have had a heart attack during surgery, and may have died.

Detecting swollen legs and feet

"I am worried that my feet are swollen at the end of the day. Is there something wrong with my heart?" Why do our lower legs and feet sometimes swell, and what can be done? Many older people notice that they develop swelling of their feet and lower legs at the end of the day. They may also note feet swelling after long car or airplane rides. This is edema (lymphedema), and it frequently frightens the individual on first noticing its presence.

Although this can be a sign of heart failure, kidney failure, liver disease, or low protein levels in the blood, the most common cause of edema in the elderly is "dependent edema" caused by some degree of venous insufficiency. It may look terrible, but it usually is not a serious problem. The "dependency" means the fluid is collecting in the lowest parts of the body (i.e., the feet, when the person is sitting or standing), as this is where gravity pulls the fluid. (Note: this condition should be bilateral, meaning in both legs.) The swelling should diminish significantly or completely after lying in bed overnight. If only one leg shows edema, a more serious local problem (such as a blood clot in the veins of that leg) must be investigated.

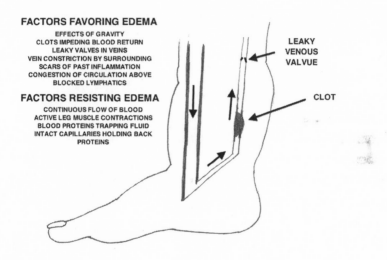

FACTORS FAVORING EDEMA
EFFECTS OF GRAVITY
CLOTS IMPEDING BLOOD RETURN
LEAKY VALVES IN VEINS
VEIN CONSTRICTION BY SURROUNDING
SCARS OF PAST INFLAMMATION
CONGESTION OF CIRCULATION ABOVE
BLOCKED LYMPHATICS

FACTORS RESISTING EDEMA
CONTINUOUS FLOW OF BLOOD
ACTIVE LEG MUSCLE CONTRACTIONS
BLOOD PROTEINS TRAPPING FLUID
INTACT CAPILLARIES HOLDING BACK
PROTEINS

LEAKY
VENOUS
VALVUE

CLOT

Fig. 2. Foot, and Risk of Developing Leg and Foot Edema. Blood enters foot via thick-walled arteries under high arterial pressure, traverses smaller arterioles and capillaries (where oxygen and carbon dioxide are exchanged, and nutrients are deposited), and returns to the heart via low-pressure veins.

While upright, or when sitting, the feet and lower legs are several feet below the height of the heart and experience the greatest gravitational pressure of blood in the veins. The veins, which return the blood to the heart, are low-pressure, thin-walled vessels (blood pressure in the veins may be only 5—10 mm/hg as compared to the much higher arterial pressure). This would seem to lead to an engineering conundrum. The pressure and weight of the blood (the hydrostatic pressure) falling downward in the vein would appear to be greater than the pressure pushing the blood back to the heart. So how does the blood get back to the heart?

This would be true if it weren't for the fact that veins have valves scattered along their length. These valves act to reduce the pressure caused by the weight of the blood above them. The height of the blood column and its weight extends only from one valve to the next. It is like going down stairs. If the stairs weren't there, and one jumped from one landing to the next lower one, we would hit with tremendous pressure and force; instead we break the impact by going down step by step.

What normally keeps our feet from swelling are these valves in the veins, the constriction of the muscles in our legs as we move about (muscle activity squeezes the veins, and there is only one direction—up —for the blood to go), and the continuous arrival of new blood to our feet via the arteries, which push the blood along. Large protein molecules in the blood also "hold" fluid from leaking out of the vessels. This is caused by the osmotic pull of these large protein molecules, which normally do not leak out of the circulation because of their size. When proteins do escape into the tissues in large amounts, or if our protein levels drop by decreased production or loss through the kidney, we lose this advantage, and lymphedema is commonly seen.

With aging, several things happen: the valves in our veins begin to leak—they have gotten old. This is called venous insufficiency. As a result, the pressure in the veins goes up, blood pools in the veins, and fluid oozes out into the tissues. When the fluid is in the tissues, and the pooling of blood in the veins increases, a new equilibrium develops with now enough increased pressure (caused by stretching the skin and tissue) to force the venous blood back to the heart. Secondly, older people usually are not as active as younger people, and with prolonged sitting, they lack the muscle constrictions needed to keep the blood flowing easily. Thirdly, many elderly have lower protein levels in the blood for a variety of reasons. There may be old damage, scarring, and inflammation in the leg that causes increased venous pressure by the obstruction at the area of injury. Lymphatics, or lymph ducts (that drain the tissues outside the blood vessels), may be blocked by swollen lymph glands, or old injury, and the tissue fluid does not drain back efficiently. A tight band of a stocking may also impede venous and lymphatic return.

The consequence of the venous insufficiency and the other problems mentioned above is that many people have considerable swelling of their feet at the end of the day. This makes their shoes tight, but is not generally dangerous. The edema is helping to keep the blood in the veins flowing. There is a danger, however, that stagnation of blood in large deeper veins can increase the risk of clots in these veins (deep vein thrombosis or DVT). We worry that these clots can break free and travel up through the heart to the lungs (or brain, if there is a "hole" in the septum separating the right from the left sides of the heart).

In general, the problems encountered with "dependent" edema (leg and foot edema caused by gravity) are: (1) increased urination at night, as the fluid from the feet gets reabsorbed, and must be eliminated—this happens with the loss of the gravitational effect in bed when the legs are elevated to the level of the heart; (2) problems walking, as a person can have many pounds of water in each leg—try to walk around all day with ten-lb. shoes and you will understand what this means; (3) if the skin is stretched too much, it can begin to "weep," or can become inflamed and infected as the germs on the surface penetrate through the pores of the overstretched skin.

The treatment of dependent lymphedema is straightforward. Keep the legs elevated on a chair or hassock, if not walking around. Wear elastic constrictive devices to apply external compression to the legs that will prevent the fluid from accumulating. Note: constrictive devices are dangerous if there is significant *arterial* disease to the legs—the constriction will decrease the pressure in the arteries further (like reducing the pressure of a garden hose by pinching it).

Many people with dependent edema in their feet ask their doctor for diuretics to "get rid of the fluid." The diuretic works on the kidney, interfering with the kidney's capacity to retain fluid. As a result of the diuretic, the kidney excretes more fluid than it normally would, and the blood will become somewhat dehydrated. Mildly dehydrated blood can absorb more fluid (similar to a saturated sponge from which some water has been squeezed out). As this blood circulates through the legs, it can pick up some of the excess fluid in the tissue. The price tag of using diuretics for removing excess leg edema is the dehydration it causes. Leg elevation or compression encourages the fluid to be reabsorbed by reducing the gravitational pull, and the blood will be slightly overhydrated. The kidneys normally have no problem in eliminating the excess fluid in the blood.

Case Example: A morbidly obese elderly woman, who has been essentially bedridden and wheelchair-bound, is short of breath lying flat in bed, and has noted marked swelling of both legs. She must wear open slippers, and keeps getting infections (cellulites) in her legs and feet. She cannot get elastic stockings large enough to fit. She is terribly depressed.

Comment: Many individuals who fit into this scenario suffer from a number of problems that give rise to leg edema. Although the edema is one of the person's major complaints, it is the consequence of many things going on, and is probably the least of her problems. Because of the massive weight of her chest, she cannot breathe easily when lying down, and had developed increased blood pressure in the arteries of her lungs due to low oxygen and poor breathing when recumbent. The right ventricle, which must pump the blood through the lungs, is unable to keep up the pressure needed, and she has "right-sided" heart failure. She developed diabetes because of her weight, which has damaged her kidneys, and is losing protein through her kidneys. She does not move, but sits most of the time in a large wheelchair. This person desperately needs to lose weight, any which way she can. With the weight loss, she would be able to breathe better, her heart would work better, her diabetes would improve, and she could be more mobile.

Pain in the legs while walking, and circulation problems

"Why can't I walk without my legs hurting?" What makes our legs hurt when we walk, and is this dangerous? Claudication is the condition where the individual complains of the legs hurting or becoming very heavy while walking, forcing the person to stop. This can become so severe that the person can walk only a few steps before the increasing pain compels him to stop. It is caused by poor arterial circulation to the feet. As the feet and legs work harder with walking, they need more oxygen and fuel (glucose). If the arterial circulation cannot keep up with the increased demand, pain (claudication) develops. This is ischemia (inadequate circulation) and ischemic pain.

For the affected person, it is helpful to note, and record, whether one leg is always worse than the other. Are the feet cool or discolored? Is this related to what shoes are being worn, or on what type of surface the person is walking? What happens with hills and stairs? How far can the person walk before the pain becomes too severe? Does stopping relieve the pain, or must the person sit down? How long must the person rest to relieve the pain?

It should be no surprise that the arteries of an elderly individual are not like those of a younger person—how could they be? Hardening of arteries and some degree of arteriosclerosis is inevitable with aging, but we have a lot of reserve and can afford to narrow the arteries significantly without noticing any problem. If arterial narrowing becomes too extreme, the feet will hurt at rest, and sores on the feet will not heal. Feet will feel better when they hang down (gravity bringing more blood to the feet) and hurt more when lying down; the feet can lose circulation entirely and become cold, discolored, and gangrenous. The best simple management of mild to moderate claudication is walking and exercising. Unlike angina pectoris, where there is pain coming from the heart that does not get enough blood, continued walking in a person with claudication will not cause a "foot attack." There is no danger of the legs falling off. Indeed, the pain of claudication is a loud and desperate scream from the legs to improve their blood supply (which the body actually can do in time with continued demand). Therefore, it is usually recommended the person walk to the point of pain, and then attempt to continue walking further. There are also some medicines available that can help, but if the blood supply to the feet is severely reduced, vascular surgeons will try to locate and relieve or bypass the arterial blockage.

There is, however, another condition, called pseudo-claudication, that can confuse the diagnosis. Here the legs also start hurting or become heavy with walking, and the person must stop walking due to the pain. In this case, however, the arterial circulation is good, but the individual, while walking or standing, is experiencing pressure on the spinal nerves that go down to the legs. It is a form of "spinal stenosis" or narrowing of the spinal canal. In pseudo-claudication, the individual does not feel better by just stopping; they must sit down to relieve the pressure on the nerves and ease their discomfort.

Large arteries, such as the aorta, can also age and develop "bubbles" (aneurysms) from weakening of the artery wall. Like a tire that develops a bulge when the tire wall weakens, the artery can develop a bulge anywhere along its length because of the pressure on the weakened wall or a tear in the arterial lining. There is a fear that the aneurysm will burst and bleed massively. Another form of aneurysm is a "dissecting aneurysm" in which a tear develops in the lining of the artery wall, "tunnels" through the wall, and may burst back into the normal arterial canal. The larger the aneurysm, the greater the risk of its bursting, and aneurysms are followed closely with scans (CT scans or ultrasounds). The aneurysm can be fixed by wrapping the bulge, insertion of an internal reinforcing sleeve, or removal by surgical resection and reconstruction of the artery. If the bulge extends to where the artery branches, circulation to those branches can be compromised.

Case Example: A seventy-year-old man (ex smoker) has noticed increasing pain in his legs when walking that has worsened dramatically the previous three months. He now finds it difficult to climb even two to three steps in the entrance of his house, and cannot walk more than a few feet. His left foot is worse than his right, and feels better when he sits up and lets his legs hang down; it hurts more when he lies down and raises his legs. He notices the left foot is darker in color, and cooler than the right. He had no detectable pulses in his feet.

Comment: This is a case of severe vascular disease in this man's feet. He was referred to the vascular surgeons and had an MRA (an MRI angiogram) of his legs, which showed diffuse arterial disease, but an area of particularly severe narrowing below the knee on the left leg. By trying to keep his legs hanging down, he was adding gravity to the arterial blood pressure and getting more blood to his foot. It is important to look for infections and nonhealing wounds in the foot or for evidence of gangrene (where tissue is dying due to loss of blood flow). He underwent a bypass surgical procedure, which resulted in a return of a weak pulse to the left foot, a warmer foot, and he eventually was able to walk further.

The agony of leg cramps

"Why do I get these severe cramps in my legs, particularly at night? They interrupt my sleep, and I am limping in pain the next day." What causes the cramps, and what can be done to prevent them? Actually, leg cramps can occur in individuals of all ages—they are not unique to the elderly. Nonetheless, they are a common problem as we age, and are the cause of many visits to the doctor. Cramps mostly occur at night, because, while lying in bed, the calf or foot muscles can go into maximal contraction without being stopped by the floor (this may also happen while swimming, but cannot happen with the foot resting on the floor).

The causes for the nocturnal cramps are not clearly understood, and may not always be the same in all individuals. The most common forms that occur in otherwise normal individuals are thought to be due to shifts in fluids and electrolytes (particularly calcium) that may change during the night when breathing and circulation alterations occur with sleep. It is important to recognize that although very disturbing, and sometimes disabling, they are not an indicator of some terrible disorder, or of a severe circulatory problem.

Various remedies have been tried over the decades, with variable success. One of the older, and still most commonly tried preventions, is taking quinine at bedtime. Quinine had been readily available for many years, but problems with quinine toxicity (heart rhythm problems, loss of platelets, and allergic reactions) forced the FDA to withdraw quinine from the market several years ago. These same problems occur when quinine is used to treat malaria, or when quinine derivatives (e.g., Quinidine) are used by prescription to treat abnormal heart rhythms. Quinine is available in quinine tonic, and many individuals drink a glass of tonic before retiring for the night as a means of preventing the cramp. Quinine tonic contains about 20 mg of quinine in an 8-oz. glass, whereas the pills contain 325 mg each. Simple mathematics tells us we would need more than sixteen 8-oz. glasses of tonic water to equal one pill—and then we might sleep without cramps, but be up all night going to the bathroom to eliminate that fluid load. Quinine has now been reapproved, by prescription only. Over-the-counter "leg cramp" pills that contain quinine are also available, but with lower quinine content.

Other medications that have been tested have met with variable proven efficacy. The most effective medicine is the calcium channel blocker, diltiazem (Cardizem). Benadryl (diphenhydramine) has also been used, but can be more of a problem in the elderly (see sleep disorders). Non-pharmacologic techniques, such as stretching, drinking more fluids (a problem before going to sleep in older people who may already frequent the toilet during the night), taking a hot bath or shower before going to bed have all had some successes and have their advocates.

Comment: I have always advised my patients to take quinine only on the evening before the cramp. This always brings a smile and the question of how can they know whether that night will be the night of the cramp. Night cramps in the legs seem to have a cyclic pattern of occurrence in most individuals. People may go months without any cramps, and then they may go into a period when they get cramps on several successive nights. I have found it helpful to recommend evening quinine (or diltiazem) for a short period (e.g., five to seven nights) after the first night of leg cramps. They can then stop the medication until they get another night cramp. If, however, the following night they get a cramp, they may take the medicine for another two to three nights and then stop. They may not get night cramps again for many months, and need no regular therapy.

Getting short of breath with doing nothing

"What does it mean to get short of breath while doing practically nothing?" A common and disturbing complaint of many elderly individuals is the development of shortness of breath with minimal exertion. With exercise, our muscles need more fuel and oxygen. In people with underlying lung disease (e.g., emphysema), the lungs may not be able to increase their breathing capacity nor keep up with the oxygen demand, and the person will feel short of breath. In individuals with underlying heart disease (heart failure), their heart may be unable to improve its pumping activity, which makes the person short of breath. In elderly individuals who have never exercised and are totally out of shape, any exertion may make them short of breath. Although very different underlying conditions, each of these problems causes the same symptom: shortness of breath. And, in reality, all of these conditions are present to some extent in all elderly.

But should older people who notice they get short of breath more easily, worry? As mentioned many times above, we are not the same as we were when we were younger. With aging, our breathing capacity drops. Further, as described earlier, our past exposure of inhaling toxins and pollutants has had its effect in decreasing lung function. Our hearts are not those of teenagers, and our general condition has deteriorated by our being less active than we were decades earlier.

Are we expecting too much from our aging lungs and heart, or is there really a problem? Since there are many older people who do not get short of breath, even with significant exercise, it shows that age alone is not the cause. The shortness of breath cannot be ignored, and if it is worsening rapidly, it may need serious investigation.

Evaluation of the complaint will require study of lung and heart function. Pulmonary function tests can evaluate how well the lungs are working and can be used as a guide to measure progress or deterioration. Inflammation in the airway of the lungs can be treated with corticosteroids and possibly antibiotics (if an infection is suspected), and reversible airway narrowing (as with asthma or asthmatic bronchitis) can be treated with bronchodilators (drugs that relax the spastic tightening of the large airways). Occasionally, muscle weakness or heart rhythm and valve problems can occur and can cause shortness of breath with minimal effort. However, there are medications and exercises that can help each and all of these conditions. Such therapies will not restore function to the extent perhaps desired, but they can improve function and breathing to a degree that allows a relatively normal lifestyle, commensurate with their age.

In severe cases, patients may require supplemental oxygen. Occasionally patients ask for oxygen at home, as they had breathed better in the hospital when they were given oxygen. The problem is that municipalities are generally worried about the indiscriminate availability and use of oxygen in people's homes. They worry about fires and explosions that may be a community hazard. Accordingly, home oxygen for therapy can be provided only if the individual has a documented need, with measurement of significantly low oxygen levels in her blood.

Case Example: An older man complains of shortness of breath with minimal exertion while walking. He is concerned about this change, and his family is worried about the significance of this complaint. On examination, he appears well and is in no distress. His EKG is normal, and his lungs are normal on examination.

Comment: This person should be examined while exercising and being stressed, not while he's sitting or lying quietly. His oxygen saturation can be measured, and can be normal at rest but be severely diminished with exercise. Heart function can be studied at rest, and at exercise with echocardiograms that look at muscle and valve function. Pulmonary and cardiac consultations may be needed.

Bothered by a chronic and recurrent cough

"I keep coughing, and it keeps me up at night." Chronic coughing can be very disturbing both to the individual and to everyone around him. It can limit his social activities, if coughing spasms occur while attending a concert, watching a movie in a movie theater, etc. It is of concern to the older person and those close to them. Could this be TB, cancer, some other infection, or caused by choking on secretions? Is this something contagious that can infect the children and grandchildren?

As with much of what this book explains, in the elderly particularly, there can be a variety of causes (some trivial, others serious) that may interact in some way to give the symptom. Sometimes the cough is due to a medicine. A specific type of medicine used for blood pressure, heart failure, and protein in the urine, called an "ACE" inhibitor, commonly causes a dry, nonproductive cough. This cough can have a benefit of reducing the risk of aspiration pneumonia, but if it annoys the individual, the medicine should be changed. Look at the medicines you are taking, and ask the doctor or pharmacist if these medicines can be giving you the cough. A nonproductive cough can also be the result of repeated reflux episodes—"a reflux cough." This type of cough is common in people suffering with gastroesophageal reflux disorder (GERD. A simple ENT examination can often suggest GERD as the cause. Postnasal drip can keep depositing small amounts of mucus into the upper airway and can produce a cough. Allergies and upper respiratory infections, similarly, can increase airway secretions, irritation, and can be responsible for coughing. Stress can cause a cough—"a stress cough." Repeated coughing itself can cause a cough by irritating the trachea. But the bottom line is that if the cough is persistent or recurrent, doesn't go away with simple cough medicines, and has not been adequately explained by a medical authority, it needs a fresh medical evaluation.

When the cough is productive, that is to say, when it produces sputum and mucus, it is due to airway irritation by fluid in the airway. This type of cough is having a value and should not be suppressed too quickly. Coughs can be a consequence of airway infection (bronchitis), pneumonia, allergy, or irritation caused by inhaling irritants. Blood clots in the large deep veins of the legs (DVTs) can break apart, showering the upstream veins with clot fragments that will flow upward with the blood and eventually get trapped in the arteries of the lung (a pulmonary embolus). These pulmonary emboli can cause coughing (even coughing up blood), chest pain, and shortness of breath. The clot will travel in the arteries of the lung (the pulmonary artery and its branches) till the artery is too narrow for the clot to go any further. It then plugs up that artery.

More commonly, coughs are not due to vascular events but to irritation of some part of the airway. The bronchi (the large air tubes in the lung) are normally lined with cells that have little hairs (cilia) that beat synchronously in a wavelike pattern. These lift secretions up and along the airway, and against gravity, to the throat. There is only one exit from the lungs, and that is the throat. If the large bronchi get scarred and distorted (as in bronchiectasis), this ciliated escalator is damaged. Secretions cannot be propelled past the point of scarring while the person is sitting or standing erect. Secretions can remain in the chest, become infected, and give repeated infections. Chronic inflammation can result in chronic coughing, bleeding into the airway, and coughing blood (hemoptysis). Occasionally, just the process of very heavy coughing can rupture lining blood vessels and cause bleeding. Smoking damages the lining cells, and affects this muco-ciliary escalator, producing a "smoker's cough."

Things to look out for are: Is there any fever, worsening shortness of breath, pain with cough or with breathing? Has there been weight loss or sweating (particularly at night—"night sweats")? Have there been any other people in the household who have had a similar cough? Any cough that has persisted for more than one week warrants an examination and chest X-rays. Tuberculosis, fungal infections, cancer, and pneumonia need to be ruled out.

Case example: An elderly woman has had a chronic cough productive of large amounts of gray sputum. She has an abnormal chest X-ray, showing inflammation, and her sputum culture grew "MAC" (mycobacterium avian-intracellular complex—"bird tuberculosis").

Comment: This is bird tuberculosis, which normally does not infect a healthy lung in a person with effective normal defense mechanisms. It is therefore not contagious to people with normal lungs. It is often seen in the elderly person who has underlying lung disease. It can be treated with antituberculosis drugs (but more drugs than usually needed to treat human tuberculosis). However, the older person with MAC pneumonia usually dies with this disease as opposed to from it. If untreated, it smolders and can weaken the individual more. The pulmonologist will often discuss the pros and cons of treatment with the patient.

The "shadow" of cancer

"I've lost some weight and feel tired. Is it possible that I have a cancer?" Older people think and worry a lot about developing cancer. Many older patients ask for total body MRIs or scans to make sure there is no cancer hiding in some dangerous place. People seem to spend a great deal of time and energy worrying about the possibility of having an undiagnosed cancer hiding in the shadows.

Although there are many types of childhood cancers and malignancies that can strike the middle-aged, the elderly are at greatest risk for developing such common cancers as colon cancer, lung cancer, prostate cancer, breast cancer, and skin cancer. Having lived a considerable portion of their years in times when the public was less attuned to environmental hazards, older people were more inclined to have smoked, to have spent many hours tanning themselves on a beach, to have consumed more nitrates, inhaled more asbestos, and were exposed more to radiation; all these exposures increase the risk of cancer. Cancer is probably the single most feared diagnosis in the general community; possibly because of the fear of the anticipated pain or suffering with chemotherapy.

Every cell in our body carries the same genes that came from the fertilized egg from which we started. What makes cells different from one another is the process of "differentiation," where most of the genetic material is "turned off" and only a small fraction of the genetic material is allowed to express itself—different portions of our genetic material expressing themselves in different types of cells. Cancer cells have lost some control of this normal behavior, and genetic material that should not be active, becomes active. Sometimes, as with cancers caused by viruses, new genetic material is added to cells that makes them malignant. Other times, genes that control normal cell behavior lose their function, in which case cancer is caused by a loss of genetic activity. Causes of change in malignant cells can be mutations, virus infections, or overstimulation by hormones. It has been suggested that our immune system developed to rid the body of abnormal cells as they periodically arise—to recognize a cell when it becomes abnormal, and to destroy it. In this view, every cancer represents a failure of the immune system to function properly. With aging, that protective function of our immune system loses efficacy.

Cancers have different characteristics of how they grow and to what organs they spread (metastasize). The difficulty of the oncologists is to find a selective (as selective as possible) feature of the cancer cells that can be exploited to kill these cells, while not injuring normal cells. As we learn more of the control mechanisms regarding cell growth and death, we are discovering new ways to combat cancer. Cancers must be able to stimulate growth of blood vessels to feed the growing tumor. If the growth of the cancer outstrips its blood supply, it would self-destruct. Therapies are now available to block this overstimulation of blood vessels. We also now are learning that many (if not all) cancers have populations of stem cells that keep feeding the cancer with new cancer cells. These stem cells may not be killed with the same cancer drugs that target the more abundant "mature" cancer cells. Much research is now directed into how to kill these stem cells.

There is also great variation in how aggressive different cancers can be. People can live well with some cancers for many years; others have more aggressive cancers, and usually have a life expectancy measured in months to only a few years. In the aged, cancer cells may grow more slowly. Routine screening for cancers should be rational. The four main cancers in the elderly for which there is regular screening are: breast cancer (with mammography), colon cancer (with colonoscopy, and checking stool for chemical traces of blood), prostate cancer (with PSA – prostate specific antigen, and prostate examination), and skin cancer (with skin examinations). Attention is now being given to screening smokers and ex-smokers with CT (computer tomography) scans of the chest for early lung cancer lesions. Since the incidence of cervical cancer decreases with advancing age, screening with PAP tests are often terminated after the age of sixty-five, provided the person had been regularly screened previously. The incidence of vaginal and vulva cancer, however, still increases with age and requires pelvic examinations. We can also test for abnormal proteins associated with ovarian cancer and for high risk of breast cancer in individuals with mutations in certain genes. We may also screen for esophageal cancer in individuals who have had abnormal appearance of their esophagus on previous examinations, by repeated endoscopies (looking into the esophagus and stomach).

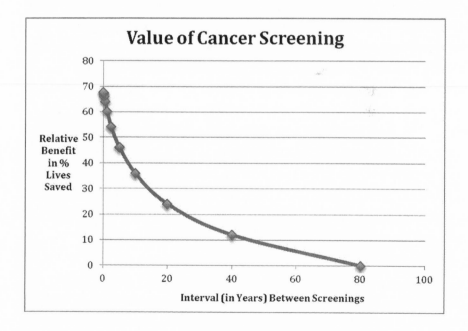

Fig. 3 Frequency of Cancer Screening Vs. Benefit

The figure above reflects the relationship between the frequency of cancer screening and likelihood of saving lives. The scales will be different for different types of cancers or conditions, but the pattern will be the same. The cost per screening test is fixed, but the benefit changes with frequency of testing. If, for example, a particular type of screening test (costing $600) were done every eighty years, the annual cost would be $7.50—an amount few would hesitate about paying—but the relative benefit would be practically none. If the test were done every ten years, the annual cost would be sixty dollars, and the rel. benefit, 36 percent; every 2.5 years, the annual cost $240, and the relative benefit, 54 percent; if performed every year, the cost $600 and the relative benefit 61 percent. What if the test were done semiannually, monthly, or weekly? Clearly the benefit shrinks with shorter intervals between testing, and the cost escalates dramatically. People with different agendas, looking at the same data, may come up with different recommendations. Someone concerned with health-care budgets may recommend setting the interval of screening at two years, believing that the benefit justifies the expense. Someone else, concerned with cancer prevention, may feel screening annually is worth the expense. For a particular patient who may be of greater-than-average risk for a specific cancer, more frequent screening is justified—but how frequent? If an insurance company will be paying for the testing (see financial issues below), someone will have to convince the insurance company to pay the extra cost of more frequent testing.

The goal of screening tests is to find abnormal cells at a time that they can be removed and before they spread. Although there is no disagreement in the medical profession that these screening tests can detect early disease and can save lives, there is some controversy as to how often people should be screened (see above), at what age to begin screening, which individuals to screen more carefully, and at what age to stop screening. Except for skin examinations, these screening tests carry some risk and discomfort. If there is a higher risk for cancer in a particular individual or family, screening should be initiated at a younger age and with more frequency. It is a matter of expected benefit vs. expected risk. If the life expectancy of an individual is less than ten years (because of an extreme advanced age or multiple medical problems), it makes no sense to screen for cancers that would have an expected survival of greater than ten years.

And again, the goal of life should not be to die cancer-free, but rather to have as much satisfaction out of life as possible. If treated early, many types of cancers are associated with dis-ease-free survival for many years; we are reminded of this in the media, when long lists of survivors, who have remained cancer and pain-free for decades, are publicized. In others, the person dies *with* the cancer, as opposed to *because* of the cancer. The cancer is like one of many types of chronic diseases, which are managed, but never cured. The concept of having a bucket list stresses the value of continuing to live one's life fully. Focusing and brooding only on one's illness interferes with the business of living.

Some individuals become terrified and irrational when they hear the diagnosis *cancer*. They feel there is no hope with the standard accepted therapy, and become vulnerable to any so-called promised cure. They may run all over the globe looking for a "cure" that is not there, but still may be advertised and offered at considerable cost. These "treatments" usually have not been proven, or have not yet been accepted by the general medical community. The person with the cancer may feel that all their money and possessions are meaningless if they die, and are willing to sacrifice everything for an unproven remedy. They feel that the benefit to them would be extreme, and worth any risk and penalty. What they risk, however, is leaving their family impoverished and in debt. They risk spending their remaining life frantically searching for something that doesn't exist, instead of enjoying their remaining life the best way they can. Oncologists do try new protocols and new therapies that have a legitimate rationale and have been shown to have some benefit with an acceptable penalty.

Case example: An older woman feels a lump in her breast while showering. She has had regular mammograms over the years, and had been told that they were normal. She is clearly worried and upset, and rushes to her regular doctor's office.

Comment: The purpose of mammography is not to prevent breast cancer, but to diagnose it early enough and before it has spread. In this particular patient, the lump proved to be benign, and the patient was advised to continue her regular mammography screening. If a new lump is felt, an ultrasound guided-needle biopsy is often performed to get tissue from this lump. If a cancer is found, a simple lumpectomy may be all that's recommended, with or without additional radiation. As a point of information, men too can have breast cancer. In men, it is generally more aggressive and resistant to hormonal manipulative therapy.

Suffering with back pain and sciatica

"I'm having pain going down my leg when I stand up; is this my back or hip? Will I need surgery?" As a practical matter, back pain usually is not a life-threatening condition, it is almost universal in the elderly, and there are many choices regarding management. Most often it is due to degenerative arthritis, where the decision of how aggressively to deal with the discomfort is based on the degree of debility the individual experiences. However, an X-ray or CT scan may be needed to make sure there is no abscess, tumor, or vascular cause for the pain that would be more worrisome. Several syndromes are associated with back pain: vertebral fracture, sciatica, spinal stenosis and radulolpathy (irritation of nerve roots exiting the spine). The causes are all fairly similar—pinching of nerves.

Why do so many of us suffer with back pain and sciatica? Our backs are often disloyal and betray us as we age. X-rays and MRI images reveal the aging of our spine and may identify problems that can accompany these changes, but images are only pictures. They cannot photograph the pain and discomfort we feel. In people over the age of fifty, X-rays will always

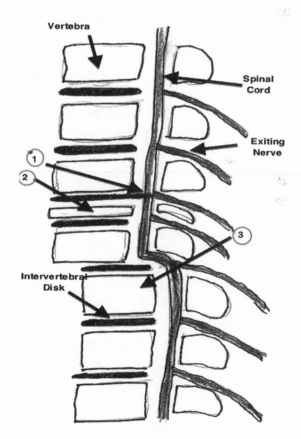

Fig. 4. Spine, showing intervertebral disks, exiting nerves, and spinal cord.

(1) slipped, or herniated disk, making contact with spinal cord and exiting nerve. (2) collapsed, or fractured vertebra. (3) displacement backward of vertebra (retro spinallisthesis), with distortion of spinal canal.

show some degree of spinal arthritis and the changes of aging in joints. People often start having backaches and arthritic pains while still in their forties. With more advanced aging, there can be slippage of vertebrae, one over the other; slippage or herniation of disks, and pressure on the spinal cord or nerve roots caused by boney ridges, herniated disk material, or ligament calcifications. When the spinal cord itself is being compressed by any of these features, it is called spinal stenosis, or central stenosis; when the nerves are being pinched as they exit through the side openings of the vertebral column (the neural foramina) it is called a radiculopathy. Although almost any part of the spine can be affected by these arthritic changes, the most common regions for developing spinal stenosis is in the neck (cervical) and lower (lumbar) regions. Individuals with lumbar stenosis will find it more comfortable walking bent forward (leaning forward creates an arc-shaped curve in the spine, which opens up the vertebral spaces and reduces the pressure on the spinal cord and the exiting nerves). As a result, they feel more comfortable leaning on a walker or shopping cart as they walk. This allows them to lean forward and shift their center of gravity in front of them without losing their balance. Others may walk with their knees bent, another way to reduce the pressure and pinching of the nerves of the back. Scoliosis, which is a sideways curvature of the spine to the right or the left, will result in some pinching of the nerves on the inside of the curve (by narrowing the neural foramina), and widening of the neural foramina on the outside of the curve.

The problem is that our spinal cord and the nerves that exit the cord traverse a space that is pretty much surrounded by the strongest bones in our body—the vertebrae. It is very much analogous to how an electrician encases major wires within a protective shield of metal or thick plastic. But the spine is discontinuous, allowing spine bending and turning, and also allowing nerves to exit from each vertebral space so that we can feel things and can control muscles throughout our body. Cartilaginous disks keep the vertebra separated from each other, keep the nerve openings spaced apart, and act as shock absorbers in the back.

We lose vertical height as our cartilage ages and dries, but our spinal cord, ligaments, and muscles, which support our vertebral column, do not shrink. As a result, muscles and ligaments lose their tension and supporting tone. With the loosening and loss of ligament and muscle tone of the spine-supporting structures, we develop greater laxity, and allow rubbing of vertebral bones together, resulting in greater arthritis in our back. When a disk slips, or arthritis occurs, there is the risk of compression of the nerves or spinal cord, since there is nowhere for nerves to get out of the way of the disk or bony growths. They cannot be simply pushed aside; they are trapped, as if they were going through a narrow canyon where rocks and boulders can crash down on them, and where there is no room for maneuvering around the obstruction. A fracture or collapse of a vertebra can produce similar complaints (see below). The result is that we often get pinched nerves, back pain, and pains going down to our legs or arms.

All sensation is felt in our brain. The brain knows where a sensory nerve (one that carries a message of what is being felt) originates. If that nerve is stimulated or irritated at the point of its origin, or is irritated anywhere along its route to the brain (e.g., the spinal cord), the brain will feel the discomfort where it believes the nerve originates. This is why there is often confusion when a person feels pain in their legs and the doctor tells them it's coming from their back (as from a slipped disk). It is also why a person can sense "phantom pain" from a limb that has been amputated. The person might not even feel any problem in his or her back.

A particular problem arises when the person has pain in the lower back and upper leg, and X-rays show degenerative arthritis in the back and in the joints of the leg. Then one has to determine the relative contribution of each problem to the total picture. If each problem is contributing equally to the discomfort, fixing one condition may not give enough relief till the other is also fixed. In young people, there generally is a single cause for a particular complaint. In the elderly, since all areas have experienced the effects of aging, few problems have a single cause, and determination of the relative contribution of each element becomes a necessity. If a principal offender can be identified, correcting that problem will have a substantial benefit.

X-rays will often disclose arthritis in the hip and knee, as well as in the spine. This should not be surprising. The older person cannot have the same X-ray picture of their joints or bones as when they were eighteen years old. Sometimes a test of nerve function is needed to determine where the nerves are being irritated. This is done with nerve-conduction tests and EMGs (a not very comfortable test, but one that is not dangerous). Occasionally, hip X-rays show no severe joint problem, and physical examination reveals an inflamed trochanteric bursitis (marked tenderness on the side of the leg below the pelvis). This bursitis can be treated quite successfully with physical therapy, anti-inflammatory medications, or injection of steroids.

Sudden severe pain in the back can be due to a vertebral fracture. With osteoporosis, the bones become weaker, and vertebrae can "collapse." If they collapse evenly, like an accordion, there is a sudden loss of height, and sudden onset of severe back pain. Sometimes the fractures are asymptomatic, and the collapsed vertebra is discovered incidentally, with an X-ray taken for other reasons. If a vertebra collapses toward the front (where it is structurally the weakest), the shape of the vertebra becomes more pie, or wedge-shaped, and a forward curvature develops (a kyphosis). With several vertebrae being so affected, the person assumes a more hunched appearance as in a "dowager's hump," or a person "bent over like a pretzel." Like with any broken bone, there will be immediate pain, which will diminish with time. Newer approaches for acute vertebral fractures now include vertebroplasty or kyphoplasty. In these procedures, hardening cement is injected into the collapsed vertebra to expand the crushed bone to its original size. In the kyphoplasty, the vertebra is first expanded with balloons before cement is injected. These procedures are still being evaluated for their long-term efficacy and value, but they can provide immediate relief of the bone pain and the pinch of the nerve. If these procedures are delayed too long, there may be some healing and scarring in the vertebra that will interfere with the success of re-expansion.

Sometimes severe bone pain in the elderly is due to metastatic cancer to the bone. Some types of cancer have a predilection for spreading to the bone (prostate cancer, breast cancer, and multiple myeloma — a cancer of antibody producing cells) —see section above on cancer. X-rays should show this problem. Bone and back pain in these conditions requires a more extensive and complex response. Radiation of the tumor lesions in the bone often can provide significant relief of the pain.

Case example: Recently I saw a woman in her mid seventies who was having such severe pain in her hip and upper leg area that she could hardly walk. She consulted an orthopedic surgeon who was a spine surgeon and who obtained an MRI of her back. He told her she needed back surgery to correct a slippage of the vertebrae (spondylolisthesis) and pinched nerves. She saw an orthopedist who specialized in joint replacements, and obtained X-rays of her hips and was told she needed a hip replacement. She was confused. She had not gotten enough relief from physical therapy, anti-inflammatory drugs, muscle relaxants, painkillers, and medications that "quiet" inflamed nerves.

I advised her that both surgeons were probably right, and that she had both back and hip problems. An EMG and nerve-conduction studies might show an irritation of the nerve roots at the spine, but would be unable to measure the relative contributions of the two conditions to her distress. Rather, she was advised to have CT-guided injections of steroids into her back to reduce the discomfort from her back, thus changing one variable. She could then see how well she could walk with her back being less painful, and her hip left untreated.

Comment: Before doing any surgery, the patient should consult the neurologist and internist, who are not vested in any one type of procedure. Activities, such as walking, are limited by the "weakest link" phenomenon. Fixing the weakest link makes the next-weakest-link the top problem. If the pain is not too severe, the person might be able to tolerate correcting only one problem.

Aching with arthritis; painful knees, hips, and shoulders

"I have terrible pain in my shoulder when I try to lift my arm. I can't cross my legs, and have terrible pain in my hip or knee when I move the wrong way—is this arthritis?" These common complaints in the elderly can make their life miserable, but are not dangerous, and will never kill the affected individual. Treatments are optional, and should be geared to how much dysfunction and pain the patient is suffering and how much they may wish to tolerate.

A good history is vital in evaluating arthritis. Is there a family history of arthritis? Has there been any trauma: falls, accidents, sudden twisting? Has there been any fever or recent infection? How long have these pains been bothering the patient, and had the individual had such pains previously? What relieves the pains, and what maneuvers make the pains worse?

Arthritis means inflamed joints. Inflammation in the joints is like inflammation everywhere. There is warmth, swelling, redness, and pain. Arthralgia means pain in the joints without evidence of inflammation. Joints can become inflamed because of trauma, acute damage to the cartilage (in joints that have cartilage), deposition of crystals of uric acid (gout), or calcium pyrophosphate (pseudo gout), hemorrhage into the joint, infection in the joint (septic arthritis), a variety of immunologic and inflammatory conditions, and chronic wearing away of the cartilage (degenerative arthritis). Anti-inflammatory medicines, resting the joint, and applying warm compresses usually help. The pattern of arthritic pain is important for diagnosis. Is it symmetrical (that is to say, affecting both sides)? Are the pains mostly in the morning, or later in the day? Usually one needs X-rays and blood tests to make the diagnosis.

In the painful shoulder, the problem is usually a result of damage to the "rotator cuff" muscles. This often happens after a fall with the arm outstretched. If the tear is only partial, exercise, heat treatments, anti-inflammatory medications, and local injections of steroids and analgesics can keep the person functioning while the tear heals. There is minimal, if any displacement of the shoulder bones. Physical therapy is important in preserving function. If the tear is complete (i.e., through and through), the shoulder bones that were held in place by the rotator muscles are more displaced, and healing will be slower. Surgery to repair the tear is an option if restoration of shoulder flexibility, strength, and range of motion are important. An MRI would be needed to see the extent of the damage. Damage to the cartilage of the shoulder—to the ligaments and tendons—will in time lead to arthritis.

The knees and hips can become damaged with falls and acute trauma, but also by the constant pressure and stress of regular daily activities. Together with the feet and back, these large joints bear the stress of walking, jumping, running, and going down stairs. As we first begin to walk, the stress of walking and the postures we assume shape the muscles in our legs and model our bones. Our adult posture and shape of our legs were fashioned by the stress on our skeleton and muscles—how the impact of walking is transmitted to these supporting structures. Once our growth has stopped, and our skeleton is complete, there is no further remodeling. If as an adult, any of our supporting bony and muscular systems begin causing problems or become painful, the effect will be felt in all supporting structures. When, because of an injury or pain, we shift our weight, trying to favor one side, or take the stress off one area, we place the weight onto structures that had not been shaped to accept that additional stress. They, in time, will complain. Arthritis in the knee or hip on one side can lead to greater impact injury and arthritis on the other side. Back problems, including scoliosis (a curvature of the spine), change the distribution of the weight to give more stress to some regions and less to others. Since the pelvis and ribs come off at right angles from the spine, a curvature of the lower spine can tilt the pelvis, raising one side and lowering the other. The hips, attaching to the pelvis, are thus angled, and one leg becomes shorter than the other by virtue of that hip joint becoming higher. Walking then becomes lopsided, as one feels when walking along a street curb with one foot walking on the sidewalk and the other in the street. The impacts are unequal and the hip and knee on one side suffer greater stress than the other. Arthritis will develop, and gait dysfunction can occur.

Occasionally, arthritis in the knee affects only a portion of the joint, where the greatest impact has been happening, and the knee angulates (usually outward). This happens most often in overweight individuals. As the lower leg points more and more outward, the force of the person's weight is transmitted more and more to the inside of the knee and foot, causing more stress in these regions. This is purely a matter of physics, transmission of force, and how the pressures are distributed. The arch will collapse if the tendon supporting the inside of the ankle tears from the stress.

Arthritis and inflammation in the pelvis can lead to pressure on the nerve bundle making up the sciatic nerve, with pain being felt down the affected leg—sciatic neuralgia. This is not really arthritis, but rather "nerve pain," as the word *neuralgia* implies.

The options available for treating pain and arthritis in these large weight-bearing joints are several. X-rays should be taken to evaluate the problem; MRI scans may be necessary if there is a question of extent of injury to the cartilage and ligaments of the knee. One can begin with physical therapy, heat, and rest (if the pain is acute). Physical therapy is very helpful, and can include pool (or aqua) therapy, where exercises are done in the water. In the water, the person weighs less, and there is less weight on the joints, but more resistance to movement, exercising the muscles more. Losing weight reduces the stress and impact on the spine and weight-bearing joints.

Medically there are anti-inflammatory medicines that can help (steroids and nonsteroidals). The anti-inflammatory medicines can be taken by mouth, injected into the joint, or applied on the outside as gels and patches. The use of canes and braces can reduce the impact on the arthritic joint by shifting some (up to 15 percent) of the weight to the arm holding the cane or crutch, or can transmit the stress around the joint to lower structures. A brace can also stabilize the joint. Braces can be as simple as an elastic bandage to a custom-made appliance. People have used acupuncture, electrical stimulation, and just painkillers with significant success. Muscle relaxants, medicines that affect nerve conduction, and anti-seizure medications can also be helpful.

If all conservative measures do not give sufficient relief and restoration of function, there is the option of joint replacement—an option that is getting more and more popular. New surgical approaches are developing rapidly, and partial replacements and joint reshaping procedures are possible. The popularity of these surgical procedures is testimony to their success. It should be restated, that in replacement of hips, knees, or shoulders, the ultimate goal is not joint replacement, but improvement in a person's life and function.

Comment: Consultation with rehabilitation doctors (physiatrists), rheumatologists, or orthopedists—can be helpful.

Suffering with painful feet

"Why do my feet hurt, and why can't I get shoes that are comfortable and stylish?" So what's causing the painful feet, and what can we do? Many elderly individuals have difficulty with their feet. Their feet hurt when they walk or stand, and they cannot find shoes that are comfortable. This happens far, far more often in women than in men. With a lifetime of wearing shoes with elevated heels, they have been throwing their weight onto their toes and forefeet for years, demanding this part of the foot bear the full weight and impact of walking. They may also have worn the stylish pointed shoes that were popular decades ago.

Many elderly develop "spurs" (calcifications in the tendons that jab into the softer tissues with the movement and pressure of walking). Some suffer with "plantar fasciitis" (an inflammation of the soft tissues in the foot), develop mini fractures of the bones of the foot, or have bunions, corns, or toes crossing up over one another, and hammertoes that cause them pain. Hammertoes occur when there is shortening of the tendons that curl the toe, resulting in a toe whose "knuckle" is bent upward. This area becomes the highest area of the foot, and can rub against the inside top of the shoe when walking. It not only can be very painful, but sores can result when the skin is eroded; infections can extend to the bone.

Some people have lost the fat pad, or cushion, located under the ball of the foot. This happens particularly in people with a high arch, and constant pressure on the metatarsals of the forefoot. Without this cushion, the impact of walking is transmitted directly to the joints of the foot. Using a soft insole in the shoe provides provides some cushioning that can help. Also, the foot can just ache (metatarsalgia), or there can be a neuroma that has developed, and this collection of nerves is being squeezed or irritated with walking.[2]

So what can you do? Some of these conditions may need surgery to correct, but most can be treated with local injections of steroids, wearing foot appliances, various types of insoles and orthotics, wearing different types of shoes, and foot exercises. In the past, the thought of wearing ugly orthopedic shoes was felt by many to be worse than the suffering caused by the foot problem. But now there are more stylish orthopedic shoes that come in colors and are more fashionable. Still, many older women chose more stylish sneakers rather than orthopedic shoes.

---

2 If the foot is not tender, swollen, or inflamed, pain felt in the foot may be due to a neuropathy (as described above, p.52).

Case Example: A seventy-year-old woman has been complaining of painful feet, and wears only sandals (even in the winter) because all of her shoes hurt her feet when she walks. She takes her shoes off at every opportunity she can, and walks around her home (or any home she visits) in stockings. She asks whether she should see a podiatrist, or a foot orthopedist, and whether she should have surgery for her bunions and hammertoes.

Comment: A good podiatrist is better than a bad orthopedist, and visa versa. It is not the professional degree that matters most; it is the individual, their approach, and their experience that matter. In this case, the woman saw both an orthopedist and a podiatrist, and both doctors gave her the same recommendation of wearing orthotics and sneakers, and, if possible, to avoid surgery—foot surgery is not comfortable, and may not relieve the problem to the patient's expectations. Furthermore, since both feet were generally subjected to the same stresses, unilateral surgery may not make the person fully ambulatory to her satisfaction.

Afraid of "collapsing" with osteoporosis

"I've gotten shorter and am worried about osteoporosis." Most shortening that elderly people experience has nothing to do with osteoporosis. As described above, our cartilage dries as we age, and we lose the "spacing height" the young cartilage in our discs and joints provided. In addition, our postures usually are not as straight, and our bending spine loses vertical height. The media has focused much attention on combating osteoporosis in women. Men, too, can have osteoporosis. People are terrified of ending up hunched over with spine deformity, fractures, and back pain. Many Americans are taking extra calcium and vitamin D to prevent getting osteoporosis.

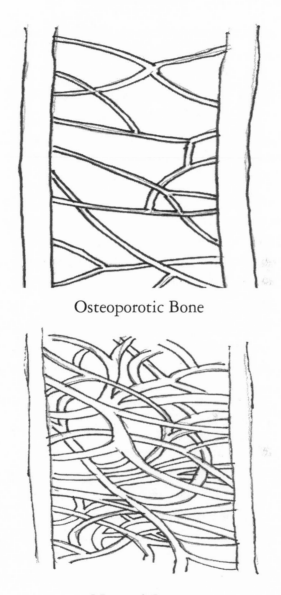

Osteoporotic Bone

Normal Bone

Fig. 5. Osteoporosis: Loss and thinning of supportive bone strengthening matrix

Bones are living tissue, with our bodies continually breaking down and rebuilding bone. As we age, the rate of bone building slows, but the rate of bone breakdown (bone reabsorption) continues, leading to an imbalance that favors bone loss. Osteopenia (which actually means diminished mineral content of bone) occurs when the mineral content has dropped below a particular value; osteoporosis occurs when the mineral content has decreased to an even greater degree, and the bones have lost structural strength. Both men and women lose bone density after twenty-one years of age. The rates of loss are similar between the sexes, but women undergo a dramatic loss of mineral in their spines (and less so in their hips) beginning with their drop in estrogen levels that herald the premenopausal period (early forties) and continuing for ten to twelve years. They then slow their rate of bone loss to that more like men (about 0.5–1.0 percent /yr.). Because women usually start off with thinner bones then men and experience the more rapid loss of bone with menopause, most of the problems of osteoporosis and fractures are seen in postmenopausal women.

Some medicines and activities increase bone calcium loss. Smoking increases bone loss in women, and less so in men. Taking cortisone (or steroids), certain anticonvulsants, and thyroid hormone increases bone loss. The diuretic furosemide (*Lasix*) and the blood thinner heparin will increase bone calcium loss. Losing weight will encourage osteoporosis. Actually having more fat improves bone density, as fat tissue makes estrogens.

Bone density measurements in women are now done routinely after menopause. What we test with bone density is bone density—not bone strength. A reasonable question is "Why should we even care about how dense our bones are?" In some conditions, such as Paget's disease, or with too much fluoride in our bones, bones can become dense, but brittle and not strong. Density is defined as the amount of substance (mass) in a volume of space. It has little to do with structural or tensile strength.

To illustrate the difference between density and strength, I frequently describe the construction of two identically sized sheds. After the frames go up, workers come into the first shed with steel beams, cement, two-by-six-inch wood studs, nails, etc. We tell them to "leave them on the floor and then get out." In the second shed, where the same materials are brought in, we tell the workers where the engineer wanted the steel beams placed, where the cement should be poured, or the studs nailed in. After they finish, they can leave. At the end of the day, if we send a beam through the two sheds, we will find they have identical density, since they have the same materials in the same volume or space. In one shed the "stuff" is organized to make the shed strong; in the other, the stuff is just lying on the floor. A density cannot distinguish between the two. In our bones, we have the same problem. Obviously, if a bone density shows there is "no stuff" in our bones, it doesn't matter how the "no stuff" is placed, we are missing mineral in our bones, and we have severe osteoporosis. The real value in bone-density measurements is in tracking the change in density over time, and how therapies are working. Bone densities are generally measured every two years.

Being told of dense bones, particularly in the spine, may not be cause for comfort. Calcifications in the ligaments around our spine will block passage of the "beam" and measure very high density. These calcified ligaments do not add to the structural strength of the spine. Severe scoliosis may cause sclerosis (a bone-thickening reaction to trauma) and produce difficulty in measuring density. Reactive bone growth may not add to bony strength, despite increasing apparent density. Unfortunately we cannot measure the strength of bones

So why don't we measure bone strength and not bone density? Measuring strength would require increasing stress on a bone till it breaks. When patients tell me they are taking calcium and vitamin D for their bones, I usually ask, "What makes you think the calcium will go to your bones?" Just putting calcium into the body does not guarantee it's going to go where the person expects or wants it to go. Perhaps it will go into a kidney stone, or calcify the arteries, ligaments, or cartilage. Calcium is deposited in areas of inflammation as part of our natural healing processes. There are many places in our body that we don't want to put excessive calcium. So how do we tell the calcium that we want it to go only to our bones? The answer is—exercise. During weight-bearing exercise, the bones ask for calcium. The bones even indicate where they want the calcium deposited to forge the greatest bone strength. And how much *extra* calcium must be added to the diet to meet our needs? As we age, we need about 1.75–2 grams of calcium daily. If we achieve that with our regular diet, there is no need for additional calcium. If we take in too much calcium, our bodies will need to get rid of the excess, and there is a risk we can get into trouble. Measuring our calcium daily intake is somewhat burdensome, and so many people just "take a little extra calcium." It should be noted that there is little dairy in the Asian diet, yet all Asians have bones, and thus demonstrate adequate calcium can be obtained from non-dairy sources. All animals with bones need calcium, and they, like humans for millennia, never took supplemental calcium pills. But they are and were more active than we humans generally are today.

Vitamin D appears to be another story. We obtain vitamin D mostly from sunlight, making vitamin D out of a pro-vitamin D in our skin. We also get vitamin D from our diet (chiefly dairy foods, in the US). This vitamin D (from both sources) is inactive, and must first be activated in our liver, and further activated in our kidneys. Having adequate vitamin D is important for bones, and low levels are associated with osteoporosis. But products of vitamin D metabolism are now being recognized as important for maintaining function of most all tissues. There are more than twenty-five different metabolic products of vitamin D metabolism now recognized that help the body with wound healing, heart disease, combating infections, diabetic control, etc. These functions suffer when vitamin D levels are too low. Vitamin D is now recognized as being much more than just a hormone involved in calcium metabolism and absorption.

In today's world, people (particularly those living in cities and living in less sunny and cooler climates) receive only a small fraction of sunlight that we believe our ancient ancestors received (particularly now, with the fear of skin cancer). We consequently don't get nearly as much vitamin D from sunlight as our forebears did. Recommended intake of vitamin D has been recently raised from 400 IUs to 600–800 IUs. Two forms of vitamin D (D2 and D3) are available, and many people are confused as to which form of vitamin D they should be taking. Both are active and helpful. Vitamin D3 (cholecalciferol) is available without a prescription, and is the vitamin form the body uses. Vitamin D2 (ergocalciferol) can easily be converted in our bodies to D3, is taken in much higher amounts, usually requires a prescription, and is often used initially to raise the vitamin level quickly. Doctors are now measuring the blood levels of the liver product (25-OH vitamin D3) as the reliable indicator of blood vitamin D3, and the levels should be greater than 30mcg/ml. It should be noted that intake of more than 4000 IUs of vitamin D (D3) can lead to toxicity. Many older people are now taking between 1000 and 2000 IUs daily to maintain an adequate vitamin D level in their blood, and monitor this level periodically.

Different types of medicines can be used to reduce bone loss by retarding bone reabsorption, and all have also been shown to reduce fracture risk. The most commonly used medicines are bisphosphonates, which reduce bone reabsorption. Taken by mouth, these medicines must not get caught in the esophagus, which is why these drugs are taken with a large glass of water, and the individual cannot lie down for at least thirty minutes after taking the medicine. Having a hiatus hernia, or gastric reflux, can give problems and require another form of administration (such as intravenous delivery). Other therapies include taking hormones such as thyrocalcitonin; an estrogen analog, raloxifene; and daily injections of a recombinant parathyroid hormone, teriparatide. A new approach to preventing osteoporosis is twice-yearly injection of denosumab. Treated bones are not normal bones, which is why they are not being reabsorbed the normal way. With the bisphosphonates, many now worry about "dead" bone, resulting from impairment of the normal bone-maintenance activity in altered bone. It is also not clear whether such bone-altering medicines need to be continued for the life of the individual. These issues should be discussed with your doctor.

But, again, what we usually care about is not our bone density or strength. We care mostly about not developing fractures of our vertebra and hips. Reducing the risk of fractures is a lot more than just taking calcium.

Case example: An eighty-year-old obese woman has been taking a bisphosphonate with extra vitamin D, and has been getting bone densities every two years as recommended. She has been having more heartburn, and had read that these medicines can upset the stomach and esophagus, and she questions whether she should continue them. In her case, the penalty of the medicine may be greater then the benefit.

Comment: Obese patients generally have less osteoporosis, as fat tissue produces estrogens, which maintain a higher bone density. People are now studying how long a person needs to take these medicines to achieve the desired effect (e.g., for the rest of their lives?). There are potential side effects from these drugs, and one can use the results of bone density as a reference to guide further treatment.

The curse of constipation

"I've always been constipated, but prunes and stool softeners are not working as well as they used to. Should I use an enema?" Although a frequent source for mockery in jokes, constipation in the elderly can be quite serious, and should not be treated too casually. Constipation may be a sign of an intestinal obstruction. It is a complaint that doctors take very seriously, and ask many questions. Fecal impaction, another cause of constipation, can require manual or even surgical disimpaction, if simple laxatives fail. If prolonged, constipation can give severe pain, and abdominal and back discomfort. It is certainly not a joking matter.

A common cause of constipation in the elderly is dehydration, and desiccation of the stool, as described above. Lack of physical activity and bed rest can put the bowel to sleep. Many medications have constipation as a common side effect.

Many elderly spend hours on the toilet. This is not healthy for the rectum or the hemorrhoidal veins, and can lead to rectal prolapse that may need surgical correction. It is important to remember that we don't need total evacuation of all the intestinal contents each time we move our bowels. This cannot happen naturally, and is unnecessary. Moving some of the stool out of the rectum will make room for more to come down and fill the space. Sitting and waiting to continue the bowel movement is not the right answer. The anatomy of our buttocks is such that when we sit on a chair or bench, our "cheeks" are closed and the rectum supported. Sitting on a toilet seat, with its open doughnut shape, spreads our "cheeks" and buttocks, allowing more pressure to be exerted on the rectum—sometimes causing bleeding from engorged hemorrhoids or rectal prolapse (the falling down of the rectum).

In evaluating constipation, it is important to know how long it has been since the last bowel movement; is this condition new;

is there any fever or abdominal pain associated with the constipation? Has the individual been losing weight? Has any new medicine been started? Obstruction usually is associated with nausea, lack of appetite, or vomiting. There may be abdominal tenderness. With fecal impaction, paradoxically, there can develop diarrhea. This is "overflow" incontinence. When the bowel is obstructed with a fecal impaction, stool coming down the bowel reaches the block, and stalls. With time it can liquefy, and pressure can build up, forcing some liquid stool to seep around the impaction, and come out looking like diarrhea. Taking antidiarrheal agents at this time is obviously the wrong approach—it can worsen the impaction. Understanding the events leading up to the diarrhea can help make the correct diagnosis. Physical and rectal examination can help identify the problem. Stool samples can be checked for presence of blood. A simple X-ray of the abdomen will show if the intestines are filled with feces.

Normal regular bowel movements need not occur every day. Some people move their bowels only once every two to three days. As long as the person is comfortable, and the pattern of bowel movements has not changed, there is no cause for alarm. Assuring adequate fluid and fiber in the diet, along with physical activity, is usually all one needs for a proper bowel pattern. Prolonged laxative use can make the bowel more dependent upon laxatives. Frequent use of enemas can irritate the rectum and make it less responsive to its normal signals. The rectum is actually a very sensitive and sophisticated part of our body. It senses when there is a need to evacuate. It tells the brain whether the distention is due to gas, liquid, or stool. Proctologists remind us of how often we don't give the rectum its proper due. Good muscle function of the rectum is needed to prevent stool leakage and proper sensing of fullness. Damage to the rectum or the nerves that control the muscles of the rectum need to be avoided.

Neuropathies can also affect the bowel. Diabetics frequently will have constipation. Low thyroid levels are commonly associated with constipation. Peristalsis (the coordinated wave of contraction that propels bowel contents along) can be affected by medicines, nerve dysfunction, or disease. There are drugs available that can stimulate or improve peristalsis.

To cleanse the bowel, in cases of significant constipation or impaction, a rectal approach is needed. Taking stimulants or laxatives by mouth, although more comfortable, can cause spasm and increased pressure in the bowel. If the impaction is severe, this increased pressure will not suffice, and the individual will only experience more pain, discomfort, and risk of bowel perforation. As with a blocked vacuum-cleaner hose, the best approach is to try to relieve the blockage from the bottom up. This can be attempted with enemas and suppositories. Manual disimpaction is left to trained personnel, but may be necessary.

Case example: An elderly woman complains each visit about her diabetic husband sitting on the toilet all day, complaining about constipation. She is asking about suppositories and enemas.

Comments: Before rushing to the use of suppositories and enemas, her husband should be examined. A review of the medicines he is taking can disclose a drug side effect as the cause. The husband needed bowel counseling. A second point in the elderly is that constipation can lead to problems with urinary control, as stool in the rectum can press on the bladder and deform it. The pain of fecal impaction can be referred to the abdomen or to the lower back. Disimpaction is never pleasant, and many elderly people regularly use their fingers to help dig the feces out, but may be too embarrassed to mention this to their relatives or their doctor.

Experiencing gas and abdominal distention

"I keep passing gas all day, and it's very embarrassing; what can be done?"; "Is there something wrong with my stomach?" Experiencing excessive belching, feeling bloated with abdominal distention, and having diarrhea are common complaints among the elderly. These symptoms can be very disturbing to your normal activities, are uncomfortable, and can be very embarrassing.

Some people refer to everything in the abdomen as "the stomach." This can lead to a lot of confusion, as the stomach is a specific organ in the abdomen. Using the same word for very different structures leads to miscommunication. It's like saying "lungs" for everything in the chest. It would be best if people used the same terminology. The words *abdomen*, or *belly* would be more appropriate terms for the space below the diaphragm. The intestines are connected to, but are not part of, the stomach, and are divided into the small intestine and large intestine.

There are a number of possibilities that can be responsible for symptoms of bloating and gas, which can be easily corrected. A common cause is a relative deficiency in lactase production, leading to lactose intolerance. Lactose is milk sugar, and its amount is independent of the fat content (e.g., there is the same amount of lactose in skim, low fat, and regular milk). The intestine normally makes sufficient amounts of an enzyme (lactase) to break down this sugar; but in the elderly, diminished amounts of enzyme may be made. Further, since the enzyme is manufactured in the intestines, whenever there is an intestinal inflammation, or more rapid transit of intestinal contents, there is less enzymatic activity per unit time, to break down the milk sugar. An excess of undigested lactose in the bowel can lead to "gas, bloating, diarrhea, and cramps."

The simplest way to determine whether lactose intolerance is contributing to your intestinal problems is to avoid all foods with lactose for a period of several days to a week (this includes all milk products, cheese, butter, ice cream, yogurt). A person can alternatively use lactose-free substitutes (soy bean), or "lactaid" products that have previously had all lactose degraded with lactase, before being marketed. If, during this trial period, no change in symptoms occurred, another explanation for the intestinal complaints must be sought.

Excessive ingestion of fruit is another common cause for bloating and diarrhea. Avoiding fruit for a week can test this possibility.

There are various foods that will generate excessive intestinal gas. Well-recognized such foods include beans, broccoli, and cauliflower. Excessive gas can also be ingested. Each time we swallow, or gulp, we swallow some air. Some individuals, particularly when they are nervous, swallow large amounts of air (aerophagia). Some of this air will be belched out, but a good amount of this air will end up in the intestine. Drinking carbonated beverages increases the amount of gas ingested. Before going for expensive testing, a prudent patient can review what it is that he or she is eating, and try some dietary changes as a tool for uncovering at least part of the problem, and as a way of managing the problem.

Other, easily remedied causes for abdominal distention include side effects of medicines, including drugs to reduce gastric acid (you can review this with your physician) and overgrowth of intestinal bacteria that produce gas as they metabolize your intestinal contents. There are a large variety of over-the-counter remedies to reduce intestinal gas that are safe and often effective.

More serious causes for abdominal pain include diverticulitis, intestinal blockage, and perforation of the intestine, or colitis, and will need a more extensive investigation. But the most severe abdominal pains occur with colic. A stone scraping through an abdominal tube causes colic. The two places where this can occur are in the bile duct (gallbladder colic from a gallstone) and in the kidney or ureter (renal colic from a kidney stone). Pain can be so severe that the person breaks out in a sweat, can become nauseated, and can pass out. Patients with colic often need hospitalization, but, if the colic is not too severe, doctors will often recommend observation, as stones can often pass on their own. Drinking lots of fluids can sometimes "push" the kidney stone along until it drops into the bladder. Individuals may need antibiotics and painkillers. Stones can be removed by dissolving them with medicines and chemicals, pulverizing them with lithotripsy by a sonic blast, or removing them by visualizing the stone via ERCP or cystoureteroscopy, ensnaring the stone, and pulling it out. The duct can be stretched with a stent or small surgical cutting at its opening, to prevent any recurrent stones from getting stuck at this site.

Case Example: An elderly woman has been experiencing increased flatulence, abdominal distention, and more "loose stool" over the past several weeks. There has been no fever, loss of appetite, weight loss, nor blood visible in her stool. She has had a "nervous" stomach in the past. She had not changed her usual diet.

Comment: Irritable bowel syndrome (IBS) rarely presents as a new symptom in the elderly, but since this woman has had these symptoms previously, it could well be another exacerbation. The absence of blood in the stool is reassuring, but should be confirmed by a more sensitive means than just her denial. A review of what medicines she is taking, or had recently taken (such as antibiotics), should be done. The possibility of an antibiotic-associated diarrhea needs to be considered.

Experiencing heartburn, reflux, and chest pain

"I'm having chest pain!"; "How do I know if I'm having a heart attack or indigestion?" One of the problems of "heartburn" is the confusion people often have in distinguishing the symptoms of indigestion from those of a heart attack. We all know of people who diagnosed themselves with indigestion and heartburn when they in fact were having a heart attack. It goes the other way around as well—people who felt they were having a heart attack, when they were having only reflux discomfort.

The brain identifies the pain according to which nerves are bringing it the message. We are made with a very sensitive sensory network on our skin (some areas being more sensitive than others). We can easily identify where we are being touched with great accuracy, and can identify things by their "feel." On our insides, we do not have the same exquisite sensory discrimination. Nerves that feel discomfort in our chest or abdomen mix with other nerves, and the brain can get confused. This is why "heart pains" can be felt in the arm, the jaw, or the chest. This is why gallbladder pains can be felt in the shoulder or abdomen. And, there are many structures other than the heart in and around the chest that can give pain: the ribs and rib joints, the breast, the skin, the aorta, the lungs, the membranes surrounding the lungs or the heart. This is why it is important to know the history, be examined, and be tested to determine more accurately what is causing the pain.

Although now recognized more frequently in people of all ages, gastroesophageal reflux disorder (GERD) seems more common in the elderly. Here, stomach contents splash upward into the esophagus and throat. This can be felt as heartburn. Frequently it is associated with having a hiatus hernia (where some of the stomach or intestine herniates up into the chest).

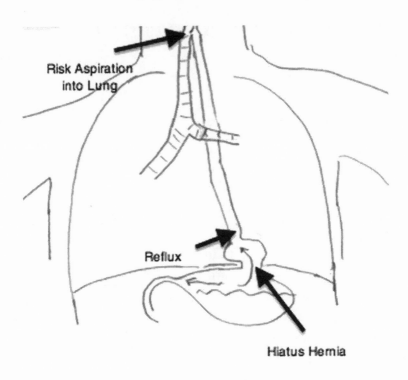

Fig. 6: Hiatus hernia, gastroesophageal reflux, and risk aspiration

The stomach acid is pure hydrochloric acid and is meant to help digest anything we eat, even the stomach of another animal (if the individual were to eat one). The healthy stomach has a protective inner lining to be able to contain such acid and digestive juices without injury to the organ itself—but not so the esophagus. Smoking, alcohol, arthritis pills, a particular kind of infection, steroids, and stress can damage the lining of the stomach. I remind patients that the presence of gastric acid was not a mistake of nature, but an advantage to survival. The hygiene and food storage of early humans was not very sanitary. The acid in the stomach reduced the likelihood of acquiring infections caused by consumption of contaminated food and water. Indeed, if the acid in a laboratory animal's stomach were neutralized, the animal can be infected with far, far fewer bacteria than if the acid was there. This becomes important for people on acid inhibitors who are traveling to places with uncertain cleanliness and purity of the water and food. It also becomes important when our food supply at home becomes contaminated. When at increased risk of food and waterborne disease, people should talk to their doctor about holding off on taking drugs that inhibit stomach acid. But nature also has a way of using new acquisitions for many purposes, and gastric acid also assists in our digestion of foods, and the absorption of iron, calcium, and vitamin B12. It reduces the risks of pneumonia and intestinal bacterial overgrowth.

If the stomach acid refluxes up into the esophagus, it can burn and partially digest the esophagus. The irritated esophagus may go into spasm, and not have a normal wave of muscle contraction; food and liquid may not go down the esophagus smoothly, and may feel stuck. Disordered function of the esophagus requires serious medical attention. There are medicines that can improve esophageal function. Then there is the risk of having food or refluxed gastric juice ending up in the lungs, instead. If this happens repeatedly it can lead to pneumonia and substantial lung disease. The esophagus itself can become scarred and develop changes in the cell composition of its lining—not a good thing. This can develop into esophageal cancer. Some people develop a "reflux cough"—a chronic cough caused by irritation of the upper airway due to the refluxed acid.

Treatment of heartburn and GERD include raising the head of the bed six to eight inches so that the entire bed is angled downward from the head of the bed to the foot of the bed. This will allow gravity to bring any refluxed gastric fluid back to the stomach, so that the acid doesn't remain in the esophagus for hours or until the person sits up. The raised head of the bed also can decrease how high up the "splash" will go when the person is lying in bed. Gastric acid that had been pushed up to the esophagus by reflux, may remain there for many hours – digesting the esophagus slowly. Individuals with GERD or hiatus hernias should never go to sleep or lie down with a full stomach, but rather allow at least two to three hours after a meal before lying down. They should not wear any constricting clothing to bed that might be putting pressure on their abdomen. Lastly, there are medicines that decrease gastric acid and are effective in stopping the esophageal burn. Non-acid reflux will of course continue to occur, but does not cause the same damage as does the gastric acid. There is controversy about how long a person should take these acid-inhibiting drugs, and whether lifelong continual suppression of acid is required. There also are medicines that relax the valve between the esophagus and stomach, and therefore increase the risk of reflux.

The acid-pump inhibitors are very effective in relieving gastric pain from a variety of causes, and are being marketed in an over-the-counter form (e.g., omeprazole, or Prilosec OTC). There was, and continues to be, significant controversy about whether these drugs should be available without prescription. The fear in the medical community is that a person with abdominal or chest pain would simply take the OTC medicine for an extended period of time if he (or she) felt relief, and thus would delay seeking medical attention and having a proper diagnosis and treatment plan made. The compromise was that the medicines would only be dispensed for a fourteen-day period, with the intent being that if the pains persisted for more than two weeks, the individual would consult a physician. Unfortunately, some individuals just go from one pharmacy to another, and keep getting these fourteen-day medication packets. For immediate relief of the distress of gastric acid, an antacid is the most effective agent. OTC medicines that are H-2 blockers (ranitidine and famotidine) suppress stimulated gastric acid for several hours.

Case example: An older person with a nonproductive cough and hoarseness was seen by their doctor and referred to an ENT specialist, who felt the individual had reflux symptoms. X-rays, taken while swallowing barium, showed a large hiatus hernia and reflux of the barium up to the throat. The patient was treated appropriately, and the cough and hoarseness resolved.

Comment: Patients usually object to raising the head of the bed with bricks, newspapers, cinder blocks, or wood, and prefer to use more pillows under their head. Pillows alone do not work. If the bed cannot be angled downward by placing 6-8 inch blocks under the legs at its head, an acceptable alternative would be to place a large wedge under the mattress. The wedge must extend the entire length of the bed, and be six to eight inches height at the head of the bed.

Trouble swallowing and aspirating food and liquid

"My father seems to cough every time he swallows." The swallowing mechanism is very complex and organized, and can get disturbed with many neurologic or muscular conditions (particularly with neuropathies). Normally, while eating and drinking, our throat is open to our lungs, and we can breathe and speak. When we swallow, or gulp, for the second that it takes, our airway is closed, and our throat empties its contents into our esophagus. We cannot talk nor breathe while swallowing. While eating and drinking, we unconsciously bring a small amount of chewed food or liquid from the mouth to the rear of our throat (when we are ready), and swallow. We raise our Adam's apple and propel what is in the back of our throat downward into our esophagus and our stomach with a gulp. If there is retained fluid or material left in the back of our throat after this gulp, it can slide down to our lungs when our Adam's apple falls back and we open the passageway to our lungs. Anything that falls into our lungs will trigger a cough reflex that can't be controlled voluntarily. Each of us have had instances of when something "went down the wrong tube" and triggered spasms of coughing. That aspiration did not cause pneumonia. We have protective mechanisms to protect us from pneumonia, including the cough.

The pneumonias that follow aspiration occur in individuals who have underlying lung or heart disease, and have been having repeated aspirations during the day and particularly at night when they are asleep (nocturnal "mini-aspirations"). In addition to what we eat and drink, we have upper respiratory secretions (such as post-nasal drips and saliva) that can accumulate at the back of our throat, and can slide down our airway. Having gastrointestinal reflux can also bring gastric materials back up to the back of the throat, and can pose a risk of aspiration. Indeed, many people with chronic lung disease have damaged their lungs repeatedly with aspirations caused by gastric reflux (see section above).

Swallowing evaluations are now more routinely used to study the swallowing mechanism. Swallowing therapists and specialists study the transit of liquids and solids through the entire swallowing procedure, and can identify specific problems that can be addressed. Too often these studies are ordered in the hospital when patients are not fully alert. They should only be done when patients are at their best.

Case Example: An older man with a past stroke has had repeated admissions to the hospital for aspiration pneumonia. A swallow evaluation showed that he routinely aspirated small amounts of thin liquids, as well as thicker liquids, when he swallowed.

Comment: Sometimes changing the consistency of the liquids with thickeners can reduce aspiration. Swallowing exercises occasionally help, but for many with severe neurologic problems, doctors often recommend the placement of a PEG tube (a percutaneous endoscopically placed gastrostomy tube). This is a small, flexible tube that is passed directly from the outside through the abdominal wall, into the stomach during an endoscopy (looking through a gastroscope that was passed from the mouth into the stomach). The PEG tube does not prevent aspiration pneumonias, as fluids still collect at the rear of the throat—it questionably reduces the risk. It does, however, allow the individual to receive adequate amounts of liquids and calories in a more timely and adequate manner; it also provides a means to deliver medications that would otherwise have been difficult to administer. The family needs to consider and discuss the value of the PEG tube with the doctor: will it be permanent—will it prolong life—will it make life better or add to the individual's value of living? These are difficult questions with no easy answer. Many people have advance directives (see below) that specifically state they wish "no artificial feedings through feeding tubes."

Another bladder infection and other urinary problems

"My urine looks darker and smells badly. Is this a urinary infection?" The color and odor of urine is not a good indicator of infection. These characteristics are more indicative of concentrated urine—a response of the bladder sensing dehydration. The more concentrated the urine, the darker and more odorous it will appear, and visa versa. Cells, minerals, or germs in the urine can cause urine to appear cloudy.

But bladder infections are very common; indeed, they probably are the most common infection seen in elderly women. The symptoms of bladder infections include some degree of loss of urinary control, as the valve controlling urination becomes inflamed and the bladder muscle itself becomes more irritated. The bladder may experience spasm, and not perform as well as when not inflamed. The most reliable symptom of a urinary tract infection

(UTI) is burning on urination (however, this is not the most frequent complaint with infection). Urinary infections can alter the state of hydration and can induce delirium in someone with an older, more fragile brain (see above). Occasionally, the bacteria causing the UTI break out of the bladder, and causes severe illness with bacteria in the blood (urosepsis). In older women the causes of bladder infections are due to postmenopausal changes in the skin surrounding the urethra (where the urine comes out), less careful adherence to the recommended technique of always wiping from front to back (difficult when a person gets overweight or develops arthritis in the shoulders), and some loss of personal hygiene. In men, bladder infections almost always indicate prostate enlargement and urine retention.

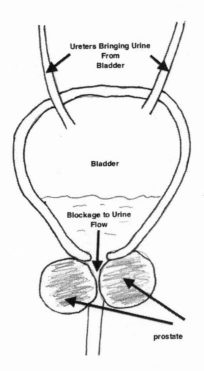

Fig. 7. Prostate hypertrophy and bladder outlet obstruction.

Any time there is retention of urine in the bladder (as when the bladder cannot fully empty, as caused by a blockage in the outlet flow of urine, a dropped bladder, or after medications that relax the bladder too much—as discussed in a previous section, p. 31) urinary tract infections are likely to occur.

It can be helpful to examine the urine for the bacterial cause of the infection. Finding the same organism repeatedly with each infection, or finding different bacteria with each infection, suggests very different problems. The first scenario means the infection was never really eradicated (as from an infected kidney stone); in the second case, one must investigate why the person keeps getting new infections.

For simple bladder infections in the elderly, the recommendation is to treat only if there are significant symptoms. Unlike younger people, where the risk of recurrent untreated bladder infections can lead to kidney disease in twenty years, we don't have this same risk in an octogenarian. The rationale for not always treating bladder infections in the elderly is that these infections are so common, that they will recur, and recur, and the frequent use of antibiotics may lead to acquiring antibiotic-resistant bacteria and to more problems than the infection alone would cause (people can develop diarrhea and colitis from antibiotic use). Taking cranberry juice and cranberry tablets may be helpful, perhaps due to the acid in the cranberry making the urine more acidic, but perhaps also due to other qualities of the cranberry that inhibit bacteria from sticking to the bladder lining. Better personal hygiene is always helpful in preventing infections. But still, in some people, the continual use of antibiotics becomes necessary if the infections are bothering the person. Referral to an urologist becomes necessary.

Individuals with urinary incontinence who are managed with adult diapers, or those who need urinary catheters will, in time, all get infections. The use of intermittent catheterization (every six to eight hours) carries less risk of infection than the placement of an indwelling Foley catheter (where the urinary catheter is left in place for an indeterminate length of time). Although this sounds terrible, patients quickly learn the routine of self-catheterization and can accomplish this task in a very satisfactory way.

Case example: After urinating, a seventy-four-year-old woman notices bright red blood in the toilet and calls the doctor in a panic. She worries about what this means. She is twenty years postmenopausal.

Comment: Many urinary infections can cause blood in the urine (hematuria). This is a form of cystitis (inflammation of the bladder) in which the lining of the bladder is so inflamed by the infection that it bleeds. Bleeding is always startling to those afflicted, and they worry about cancer (which can also cause bleeding, as can stones, inflamed diverticulum, etc.). Many doctors will culture the urine, treat with antibiotics, and hold off referring to the urologist unless the bleeding continues.

Aspects of infections and fever in the elderly

"I'm sick with a cough and feel feverish; can you give me an antibiotic?" This is a common phone complaint from a person who feels sick and wants an antibiotic. They have had many infections in the past, and had always recovered within several days after taking an antibiotic. It is cold and nasty outside, and they are reluctant to get dressed and come to the hospital, clinic, or doctor's office. They would much prefer to stay in bed, drink tea or soup, and take an antibiotic. What's wrong with telephoning in an antibiotic? The problem is that there is no quick satisfying answer to this person's question.

Fever should not be used as the prime indicator of infection in an elderly person. Fever is often diminished in the elderly. The diminished fever is not a good thing, as fever is part of our natural defense against infection—it helps us kill germs. Fever is not a response of the germs to hurt us. When the elderly were younger, and raising their school-aged children, the older person typically used the amount of fever as the indicator of how sick their child was from any infection. Schools encouraged this, and used the degree of fever as the principal determinant of whether a child should stay home, or be allowed to come to class. The effect of that attitude is that older people still use the presence of fever as the prime barometer of the presence and severity of an infection: the higher the fever, the sicker you are. This is an erroneous concept, particularly for the elderly, where an infection can fail to stimulate a fever. Indeed, a subnormal temperature is more indicative of a severe infection than is fever. Fever results from shivering. With less muscle mass (see above section on changes in body composition with aging) we have less muscle shivering, and older people can be without fever (afebrile), despite severe infection. Slower metabolism can also contribute to development of less fever. Since fever is not always a reliable indicator of infection or inflammation in the elderly, we need to look for other parameters. The additional parameters of infection and inflammation include redness, pain or tenderness, and swelling in inflamed areas. These remain good indicators of inflammation in the elderly. Finding an elevated white blood count (WBC) is a good laboratory marker of infection or inflammation; the rapidity of the rise in WBC can be slower with infection in the elderly than in younger people.

Infections are common, and people have survived infections of various types for tens of thousands of years—way before the discovery of antibiotics. Our bodies are equipped with many natural defenses to fight and prevent infections. Understanding the significance of the infection is important: is the infection the problem, or is it the symptom of some other process?

Infections are, at least potentially, curable, and therefore they need serious consideration. Any time there is an unexplained change in the function of an elderly individual, the possibility of a new infection should be entertained. Why is the infection happening when it does? Frequently investigation as to the cause of the infection leads to the discovery of an underlying condition that was partly responsible for, or contributory to, its development. In the past, as well as now, infections can be the terminal process in an older person dying from cancer, heart failure, or kidney or liver failure.

It was once taught that pneumonia (infection) was a friend of the old man. That infection would take away the old and infirm quickly and painlessly, thus saving them from the "cold degradations" that the underlying illness would impose. This was the teaching of Sir William Osler, the most distinguished physician at the end of the nineteenth century. In those days, there were no antibiotics, and Osler could well afford to be philosophic about the good qualities of something that he was powerless to stop. In today's world, with antibiotics, physicians have to understand whether the infection is coming as a friend or as a foe: Do we welcome the infection, or fight it with whatever means we have available?

For influenza, specific antivirals (not antibiotics) should be started within forty-eight hours of the onset of the infection. How then does the individual (or the doctor, for that matter) know what to do? Not prescribing the antiviral as a response to that first phone call may delay treatment beyond this window. The way the illness developed is a good clue to its cause. Influenza was not called "the Grip" for nothing. It typically "grips" the affected person suddenly and severely. Before calling the doctor for an antibiotic, collect your thoughts and think about how the condition developed. The doctor might consider if this infection is occurring during the midst of a community epidemic. Is there anyone else in the household who has or recently had similar symptoms? Does the person have a cough, nausea, diarrhea, burning urine, etc.? The patient should "listen" to their body. If they feel very weak, ill, short of breath, sweaty, they should be seen and examined, and not just take antibiotics prescribed over the phone. If there is a holiday coming up, there may be no one available to help them for days if they delay seeking medical help. If there is no one at home to help take care of them, they need help. At a clinic or hospital, they can be examined, have their blood, sputum, or urine tested, get X-rays, a rapid influenza diagnostic test, and then treated more appropriately.

As discussed below, there are significant problems associated with the indiscriminate use of antibiotics. Doctors don't like being the bad guy, and may empathize with the patient, but their training teaches them that infections in older people can be serious, and many noninfectious conditions can masquerade as an infection. Expediency should not be the reason for taking or not taking antibiotics or antivirals.

Since the end of World War II, widespread use of antibiotics became common. The public quickly developed overconfidence in what antibiotics can do. Patients often ask for "a strong" antibiotic, as if doctors were in the habit of using "weak" antibiotics, unless otherwise directed. Any antibiotic that eradicates the bacterial infection is strong enough. In time, with antibiotic use, bacteria that had mutated to make them resistant to these antibiotics were genetically selected; they could survive and grow while the antibiotic killed off their competition. Newer antibiotics were needed to treat bacteria that were resistant to the older antibiotics; bacteria then developed mutational changes to make them resistant to the new antibiotic and we entered the next cycle of trying to make newer antibiotics that can treat infections with these resistant germs. This pattern exists today. Hospitals are wonderful places for these resistant germs to emerge, since there is a lot of antibiotic pressure suppressing their competition.

A particular problem with "broad spectrum" antibiotic use is development of a very serious colitis caused by *C. difficile*. This germ is very common, but lacks the competitive edge to cause a colon infection, unless the broad spectrum antibiotics destroy the "good germs" normally inhabiting the colon. In the elderly particularly, *C. difficile* infections are common after antibiotic use, may be recurrent, and may be very difficult to eradicate.

What we have learned in the "age of antibiotics" is that antibiotics alone cannot always cure the infection. What antibiotics do is assist the patient's defenses in recovery, these same defenses that kept our ancestors alive during their nonfatal infections in the pre-antibiotic era. When individuals have such weakened defenses that they cannot mount an effective response, no antibiotic may be able to cure the infection. This is when doctors tell the patient and family that the bacteria may be "sensitive" to the antibiotic, but the infection is resistant. Abscesses are an example of infections that must be treated with drainage, as antibiotics alone are usually ineffective. An infected prosthesis (such as a joint replacement or metallic heart valve) is another type of infection that usually needs surgical removal of the infected device to clear the infection. Since the advent of HIV infections, the importance of host defenses became apparent. This is why patients with malignancies, being treated with chemotherapy, are so prone to serious infections, and why an infectious disease is so often the terminal event in debilitated and severely ill patients.

The "normal defenses" against infection are: (1) an intact skin barrier, keeping the germs on the outside, and keeping our insides sterile. In many elderly, breaks in their more fragile skin occur, and germs can gain entry into the body. Furthermore, hospitalized patients frequently have their skin pierced with needles, as for an IV; their bladder penetrated with a catheter; or the lungs invaded with suctioning or breathing tubes. (2) Effective white blood cells with a good circulation to bring the battle to where the germs are located. In the elderly, white cell function diminishes, and the circulation may not be adequate to bring the cells, increased oxygen, antibodies and antibiotics to where the infection rages. (3) Fever, inflammatory proteins, cough, and an adequate immune response all protect against infection. In the elderly, each of these defenses can be diminished. I often remind patients that fever, cough, and inflammation were responses nature provided us to fight infections; they are not part of the bacteria's arsenal to fight us. Unless the fever and cough are disturbing to the patient, there is no compelling reason to suppress these natural defense mechanisms. It should be emphasized that fever, although usually due to infection, is actually part of an inflammatory response, and can be seen in noninfectious inflammatory states. Fever can also be caused by medications, by death of tissues or cells after a loss of blood supply, by arthritis, or by any significant inflammation. As a point of information, *fever* is the correct term to use for an elevated temperature. Demonstrate your sophistication by not using the word *temperature* when you mean "fever." Every physical thing in nature has a temperature.

Case example: A seventy-five-year-old woman feeling "sick" and nauseated called the doctor's office asking for an antibiotic. She was told to come to the office for an examination, where it was discovered she had localized tenderness in her abdomen, had a fever of 100.5 F., and a rapid heart beat. A CT examination of her abdomen revealed a diverticulum (an out-pouching in the wall of the colon) that was infected and had ruptured; she was sent for emergency surgery, and did well postoperatively.

Comment: Many things may cause fever and discomfort. Unless the doctor knows the older patient well and is confident that the problem is due to a mild infectious disease, the patient should be seen and examined. Long-distance treatment of infections is risky and not advisable.

Seeing "ugly" lesions on your skin, and hair thinning

"How worried should I be about these skin discolorations?" This is a common complaint, and aside from the cosmetic issue, most people are concerned about skin cancer. Should a dermatologist see all skin lesions? With financial worries, most people hesitate in seeing more doctors. Even with insurance, it's going to cost money.

Elderly people routinely get "age" spots. These discolorations are usually lentigenes, which carry no dangerous potential. If they bother you, you can have them removed cosmetically, but you will get new ones. Years of chronic sun and cold exposure leave the skin dry, tight, and with sun damage. There can be ugly rough pigmented raised blotches called keratosis. With aging, the skin gets thinner and blood vessels in the skin are more fragile, resulting in more "black and blue" bruises (called ecchymosis, pronounced *ek-ee-mo-sis or ek-ee-mo-sees for pleural*) with minimal or no trauma. People taking warfarin (Coumadin), aspirin, or corticosteroids will increase the number, size and frequency of these ecchymoses. These lesions are not dangerous, although their appearance is frightening and disturbing. Small little blood vessels in the skin (called capillaries) can become distended and clotted, appearing as "large blue spiders" in the lower legs.

With aging, cells that normally police our skin, by percolating through the skin and removing abnormal cells and things that don't belong there, lose functional activity, and are less numerous. This may be a reason for more skin cancer in the elderly. And lastly, wound healing in the elderly is slowed. Most of these conditions are benign and do not require any specific treatment other than cosmetic camouflage. If the skin discolorations keep enlarging, it is cause for concern, and the individual should be examined.

People worry about skin cancer, and are concerned about non-healing wounds on their bodies, recurrent sores, or "funny" discolorations on their skin. They may try to cover these spots with makeup. Often the children notice these "lesions" and bring their parent to the doctor's office. The diagnosis may be obvious, as with shingles (zoster), thrush (a yeast infection), or gangrene, but often, a dermatologist is needed to make the diagnosis. If a skin lesion is painful, changes its appearance, bleeds, persists for weeks, or comes back in the same location, there is greater concern.

Thrush is typically seen in the creases of skin, where the Candida fungus enjoys a warm, sweaty, and moist environment. There is a distinctive strong odor that comes from the lesion. Patients usually try to hide the lesions, but the skin can "burn" and hurt. Most commonly cutaneous thrush develops under the breasts, in the groin, armpits, or under fat-folds in the abdomen of obese individuals. Treatment with antifungal medication works, but to prevent recurrence, the skin needs to be kept dry, and various drying and antifungal powders are used. Thrush can also occur in the mouth, particularly if the mouth is dry from mouth breathing and decreased saliva production. With oral thrush, the tongue is coated with white to yellow-white patches that can be seen on the inside of the cheeks and in the back of the throat. This type of mouth/throat thrush can make swallowing difficult and can affect the appetite and eating habits of the afflicted individual.

The skin can become excessively dry, and can itch. The drying can be due to the use of soaps that remove natural oils from the skin, excessive washing, medications, dry air (as in winter-itch), dehydration, and sun damage. With aging, less body oils are made, and our skin is more prone to drying. Skin lubricating creams and oils are readily available without prescription. Itchy skin can be a symptom of a more serious underlying condition, such as lymphoma, and if it doesn't respond to lubricants, a dermatologist should evaluate it.

Aside from "ugly" age-spots, a common dermatological complaint of older women is hair thinning and hair loss (alopecia). About 30–40 percent of older women have some noticeable hair loss, and many try to disguise this by various cosmetic maneuvers. The most common cause of hair loss in older women is an increase in levels and activity of the male sex hormone, 5-hydroxy testosterone (5-HT), and decreased estrogen. Women make testosterone from estrogens by means of a simple enzyme action (it can go the other way as well – men can make estrogens from testosterone). In older women, elevated 5-HT levels may lead to "male-type" baldness (as well as increased hair growth on the face). While this is not dangerous, it often is a source of distress and embarrassment. It can often be managed with application of "over-the-counter" minoxidil, rubbed into the scalp. There are some prescription pills that can be taken to reduce 5-HT, and stronger lotions that can be applied. If the hair-loss doesn't stop, or becomes more noticeable, a visit to a dermatologist is advisable, since other, less common conditions can cause hair loss.

Case example: An elderly woman is found to be wearing excessive makeup on one area of her face, and this had been noticed by her daughter who brings up the lesion to the doctor during a routine visit. The patient tries to dismiss the skin lesion, as she has had many skin lesions during her life. She had had significant sun exposure when she was younger.

Comment: Skin cancers are a heterogeneous collection of malignancies. The most common are the basal cell cancers (or epitheliomas). These are a result of sun exposure; they grow slowly and never metastasize. Squamous cell carcinomas are more invasive, and have a greater likelihood for spread. Lymphomas can invade the skin, particularly in individuals with immune deficiency. The most feared skin cancer is melanoma, a cancer originating in the pigmented skin cells—melanocytes. Melanomas can spread almost anywhere in our body if they are not removed very early. Since our eyes also contain these pigmented cells, melanomas can also originate in the eye.

Why do we get pressure ulcers?

"I'm lying in bed all day, and have pain around my backside. People tell me there's a sore down there." Pressure sores can be avoided. They are due to a loss of blood supply to an area of skin and muscle caused by prolonged pressure. Press your finger forcefully against your skin or fingernail, and you will see the skin blanch underneath the pressing finger. What you have done is squeeze the blood out of the capillary blood vessels that feed the skin. Prolonged sitting, lying, or being in any position for over two hours, will damage the underlying skin and tissues. The tissue of the skin is being deprived of blood and oxygen. The damage can cause simply reddening of the skin to death of cells and loss of skin over the wound. With more prolonged deprivation of blood, a deep ulcer going down to muscle and deep tissue occurs. Once the skin is broken, germs enter, and an infection occurs.

Conditions that lead to immobility may be: Parkinson's disease, stroke, restraints, weakness, dementia, sedatives, and prolonged bed rest during hospitalization. Dehydration is bad for skin resistance to pressure. A person who is immobile must be turned or repositioned at least every two hours, or have her weight spread over a greater surface area, to prevent tissue and skin damage. The location of the pressure ulcer will depend upon how the person spends most of their time (e.g., lying in bed or sitting in a chair). The areas experiencing the greatest risk of pressure damage are at the base of the spine (sacrum) heels of feet, and shoulder blades. If one observes people as they sit or sleep, we all briefly and regularly change our position (even if only for a second). That shift in position lets blood refill the blood vessels of the skin. Older people usually have less subcutaneous fat. Thin people, and people who have lost much of the fat under their skin, are particularly vulnerable (less fat means less "padding"). That fat padding spreads and absorbs the pressure and stress of the person's weight. Additionally, sheer forces, as encountered when pulling the person against the bedding, traumatizes the skin. Incontinence leaves the skin soiled and wet and damages the skin. The skin should always be kept clean and dry.

When a pressure ulcer develops, the single most important way to manage the sore is to relieve the pressure being exerted on it. This lets the blood and healing factors back in. In treating an infected skin ulcer (a decubitus ulcer), superficial cultures, taken from the surface of the wound, may not reflect the makeup of the germs that are infecting the deeper tissues. If the ulcer becomes deep and large enough, the infection can extend down to the muscle and even the bone, making wound repair difficult. There are no skin cells at the lower depths of the ulcer that can generate new skin. Surgeons will remove all dead or infected tissue, to get down to healthy tissue. They can then graft normal skin and muscle to the damaged area to allow new healing. In an analogy, one can only plant a good lawn on fertile, well-watered soil. But again, pressure must be relieved to allow a normal blood supply.

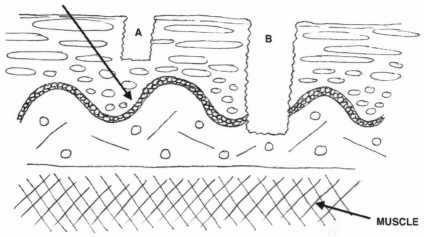

GROWING LAYER OF SKIN CELLS

A

B

MUSCLE

Fig. 8. Skin ulcers. The area between the muscle layer and the growing layer of skin cells contains the vital blood vessels that feed the skin. A shallow ulcer, such as ulcer "A," will easily heal without a scar, as it does not disrupt the growing layer of skin cells. A deeper ulcer, such as "B," can only fill in with skin cells coming from the sides. A deeper ulcer (not shown) that extends through the muscle layer to the bone beneath may require more extensive surgical repair, and removal of all dead or infected tissue, to heal.

Case example: A ninety-two-year-old man was recently seen with a large skin ulcer over the Achilles tendon of his left foot. The ulcer was covered with a thick gray material, and was not bleeding. The individual normally sat for hours with his left foot and heel pressed against a bar on his wheelchair.

Comment: The person above needed evaluation of the arterial circulation to the foot, as trying to close the ulcer would require a good blood supply to the leg and foot. The circulation was diminished, but considered adequate to proceed with scraping away the gray material ("granulation tissue") till the clean under tissue was exposed, clean, and bleeding. The plastic surgeons could then close the wound. If the circulation had been shown to be inadequate, improving the blood flow to the foot would have been needed. A decision had to be made in this elderly man, of whether "fixing" this ulcer, or leaving it covered with bandages, would make his life better. Since he had pain, he wished the ulcer to be "fixed."

Those annoying drying conditions

"Why do my skin, my eyes, and my mouth feel so dry?" Many older people suffer with dry eyes and a "sicca," or dry syndrome. In the sicca syndrome, there is also drying of the nose and mouth. It is uncomfortable, and when it involves the skin, there is usually itching; when involving the eyes, there is burning; and when involving the mouth, there is that "pasty" feeling. So what does it mean, and what can we do about it?

Excessive drying can be due to dehydration, overuse of diuretics, taking any one of a number of medications that have drying effects, some inflammatory and autoimmune conditions, and exposure to excessively dry air. Dry eyes can cause eye discomfort, corneal irritation, and can result in the individual trying to keep his or her eyes closed (dry eyes feel better with the lids closed). Keeping the eyes closed, of course, is an invitation to falling asleep. Dry eyes can easily be diagnosed by the ophthalmologist, and usually improves with artificial tears and eyedrops. However, this is most often a chronic condition that needs long-term or lifelong treatment. Production of tears can be measured after instilling a minor irritant into the conjunctiva and measuring tear production using a wick of filter paper. A biopsy of the mucous membrane lining the mouth can be easily done, looking at the microscopic appearance of the mucus-producing glands. Such testing can result in disclosure of what conditions are causing the drying, and how best to treat the underlying condition.

With a dry mouth, people suck on hard candy. Sour citrus candies can help stimulate saliva production. However, it may not be enough. Drinking water, or sucking on ice cubes, offers only immediate and very transient relief while the water is in the mouth. There are products that more closely resemble saliva, with a "mucuslike" oiliness that can be purchased over the counter (saliva substitutes), that are more effective. A dry nose is helped by saline nasal sprays, which are readily available over the counter.

Dry skin is common in the elderly, and can cause itching and flaking (see above). On the scalp it appears as dandruff. As mentioned above, aging itself is often associated with drying of the skin. Our total body water content decreases. Using an oil-based soap, one that has lanolin, or a skin softener is preferred to using a pure soap. Using moisturizers and oils are helpful. Use of humidifiers to keep the air we breathe moist during the winter season is helpful. Previous generations used pans of water on the windowsill—today we have efficient and safe humidifiers for winter use.

There is a psychiatric condition in which people "pick" and mutilate their skin to the point of developing sores in all the areas they can reach. The sores themselves are itchy, and can become infected; the cycle continues. Chronic diffuse severe itching, and drying may be a symptom of more serious conditions, and a dermatologist should be consulted. A biopsy may be needed to help understand the problem.

Case example: An older woman complains of dry, itchy skin over most of her body. She is constantly scratching and developing sores as she excoriates and mutilates her skin with the scratching.

Comment: Irritation from wools and allergies to fragrances in soaps and detergents that linger in her clothes should be considered. Chronic scratching alone can irritate the skin and perpetuate the itch. She should be advised to try changing her soap, using body creams—and be referred to a dermatologist if these are not helpful.

Unhappy with your weight

"I can't seem to lose weight, and I don't like what I look like." As previously described, weight gain is common as we get older. A healthy older person has to work very hard to prevent weight gain. Even maintaining one's weight is seen as "getting fatter," since as we lose height, we package the same weight in a shorter space, and we often bend forward. Also, as mentioned above, our body fat content increases with aging, while our lean body mass decreases.

In everyone, weight change is a reflection of number of calories in, and number of calories expended. As our metabolism and activity slows with aging, we don't "burn" as many calories as we did when we were younger—but we still eat. And eat we do. Every social gathering seems to be centered on consumption of something with calories—usually lots of calories. If weight loss is important, that person must try to decrease the calories consumed, while exercising more and burning more calories.

As a practical point, one must distinguish whether the excess weight is unattractive to the individual, or is really unhealthy. Although the goals of life should not necessarily be to die skinny, being overweight does carry significant medical risks. Diabetes is clearly related to obesity. Many people develop diabetes with weight gain, and find the diabetes resolves with weight loss. All diabetes is associated with increased risk for vascular disease, neurologic problems, vision changes and cataracts, renal disease, and decreased resistance to infections. Obesity is also associated with arthritis of the larger weight-bearing joints of the hips, knees, and back (joints that have to bear the extra burden and impact of the weight). A peculiar bursitis below the knees (Anserine bursitis) is rarely seen in non-obese individuals; with anserine bursitis, the patient often feels the pain in their knees when they walk, and assume it to be arthritis. Like bursitis elsewhere, it can improve with physical therapy, local injections, and anti-inflammatory medications. Hypertension is associated with obesity. With obesity, it can be harder to exercise, and people often become more sedentary, leading to greater weight, and the vicious cycle of further weight gain. With morbid obesity, maintaining personal hygiene becomes a problem.

In people suffering with diabetes, weight gain is particularly a problem, as most medicines used to control the blood sugar can make the person hungry. A drop in blood sugar stimulates hunger. This, too, can lead to a cycle of weight gain, worsening diabetes, more medicines, more hunger, and more weight gain.

Weight loss and anorexia is also common in the elderly. Families and older persons worry about weight loss and fear its cause and significance. When feeling sick, or after injury (including surgery), nature tells us not to go out foraging for food, but rather to hide in a cave or under our blanket until we feel stronger. This had great survival value. Loss of appetite is frequently caused by depression (which can cause some people to eat more and others to stop eating). With advanced dementia, people can forget to eat, and can even forget how to eat. They may not know what to do with food in their mouth, and spit it out. Problems with swallowing or stomach irritation can cause loss of appetite. Oral and dental problems can lead to difficulty chewing. Fecal impaction or obstruction will cause nausea and weight loss. Occult malignancies and infections can cause anorexia. Medicines that cause nausea will also cause loss of appetite. Fear of aspiration and choking can cause anorexia.

Although there are a variety of appetite stimulants, an investigation as to the cause of the loss of appetite is warranted. This may include a review of medications recently started and a referral to a gastroenterologist for possible endoscopy (looking down into the esophagus and stomach for a visible cause).

Case example: An eighty-year-old obese, diabetic man is requesting referral for bariatric surgery (banding of his stomach). He meets the obesity criteria of BMI (body mass index), and knows an individual who had lost considerable weight with gastric banding. He is concerned his insurance company may not approve the surgery, and is asking for a letter of necessity.

Comment: The insurance company will rightly ask what other measures had been tried by the individual to lose weight. The TV program The Big Loser *publicizes there are alternative ways to lose weight. Most people are looking for a quick fix, a pill or surgery for weight reduction, rather than the work and effort of exercise and eating restraint.*

Hardships of living disabled

Events happen which sometimes lead to disability: a fall, an accident, a loss of vision, a stroke, a surgery gone bad, a worsening of a degenerative disease—suddenly the older person can no longer take care of herself the way she previously had. Newly disabled older people are no longer able to help their spouse (if they have one), and now need help themselves. The family is in crisis, and goes into crisis mode. "Can the affected person still live in the same facility in which they had been living?" "Who is going to take care of them? Who do they call for help? Can they afford the cost of additional help? Who is going to take care of the bills and everyday needs, like shopping, cleaning, food preparations, and the hundreds of things that pop up and need attention during the normal day?" If they have children, family members now feel the pressure of "the sandwich generation." They need to care for their children as well as for their parents. The entire family is affected by the disability.

Fortunately we now live in an age where society has accepted the rights of the disabled person to live as normal a life as possible. Laws demand public places be "handicapped-accessible." Public buses, trains, and airplanes can be accessed by the handicapped. Self-opening doors and elevators have been installed in public buildings to make them accessible. Sidewalks have "cuts" at corners to remove the obstacle caused by a curb. Street crossings in cities are now giving advance warnings of when the light will change, which limits the risk of getting caught in the middle of the crossing when the traffic changes direction.

If the person has been disabled for a long time, they probably have already established a routine that allows them to function relatively comfortably in their usual environment. But if the disability is a new or sudden event, the family crisis mushrooms. Most people start by consulting their physician. The older individual is usually in a hospital or medical facility when the disability occurs, or immediately after the event. In the facility, there is a staff of individuals to assist and counsel the family and the patient. There may be a rehabilitation service at the hospital to begin the rehabilitation after the acute injury is stabilized.

Disability comes in many forms. There is mental disability— from dementia, to depression, to psychiatric—that interferes with "normal function." There is physical disability from loss of vision, hearing, moving, breathing, and pain. Each type of disability needs its individual evaluation and attempts to minimize the impact of the problem on the individual's life.

A sudden disabling event, such as a stroke or loss of a limb, will always cause deep depression. Life will never be the same as it was before the event. Eventually, the patient and their family must get beyond the anger and depression, and get on with living the best life possible. Psychologist visits are a routine part of a rehabilitation program.

Patients often don't understand the difference between acute rehabilitation and sub-acute rehabilitation. In an acute rehabilitation facility, the person is expected to be able to participate at least four hours/day in an active program. If their concentration, mind, or body is not up to this rigorous program, they will be considered as "inappropriate" for acute rehab, and transfer to a sub-acute facility will be recommended. In a sub-acute facility, only one hour/day of exercise is needed. Further, in an acute care facility, there are a list of conditions and performance levels, which must meet admission standards; if these criteria are not met, the person is not eligible for admission. The insurance companies, who pay the bills, and withhold payment if their criteria are not met, impose these regulations. It is not unusual for patients who are not yet ready for acute inpatient rehabilitation to go initially to a sub-acute facility to gain strength and endurance, and later be admitted to an acute rehab facility when they become able to participate at the four hours/day demand. Individuals who fail the admission criteria to the acute rehabilitation facility of their choice, and are told that they should go to a sub-acute facility, often feel despondent, as if they had failed some important examination or test. They plead for reconsideration, as if asking for a passing grade. It should be explained that a sub-acute stay is not forever (usually lasting only a couple to a few weeks in duration), and the level of care is appropriate and geared for their level of function.

At the rehabilitation facility, there are people and services that can assist in modifying the home of the disabled individual to allow them to return and function in their own residence. These services can also be provided in the community by agencies such as the visiting nurse services or other local nursing services. The goal is to allow the disabled individual to function independently as much as possible in their preferred living environment.

Once home, even with modifications to the home, adaptations to the normal activities of living need to be made. Simple things take a lot more time to be accomplished. Advance planning for every day's activities needs to be done. Until a new routine is established, the disabled individual will need a lot of handholding and support.

Case example: After a fall and hip fracture, an older woman was sent to a sub-acute rehabilitation center for recovery. Her walking progress was slow, as initially she was not allowed to put full weight on her operated leg. She had developed edema in the affected leg as well as a bladder infection in the hospital. She wanted to go home and sleep in her own bed.

Comment: After a hip fracture, there are risks of developing clots in the veins of the leg, edema in the leg due to the swelling and inflammation around the area of surgery and fracture, and urinary infections from the urinary catheter that is always inserted. Afflicted individuals have to sleep with a wedge between their legs, to keep the hip in the correct anatomical position. This patient's life was totally altered as a result of the fall. With time, she adapted to the routines and the new ways she had been taught to dress, walk, and move. She returned home when she was better able to care for herself.

Important Family Concerns

Few live alone and in a vacuum, without involvement of concerned family members. The problems encountered with aging affect families, not just individuals. All aspects of living come under scrutiny. How well can the aging individual manage his own affairs?

Managing his or her own finances and paperwork is an expression of independence, and is good for the older individual. It provides a brain challenge, keeps the individual involved in life's activities, and provides a sense of competency. However, the challenge sometimes can be too great, and mistakes are made. Often the legalese of official or business papers arriving by mail is too confusing for anyone without a law degree to decipher. Sometimes grown children fear their elderly relative has been "duped" into subscribing to "clubs" or donating money to fraudulent charities. Elderly people are vulnerable to scams. There may be a great temptation for the adult child to step in and try to manage a parent or grandparent's finances and papers. This can escalate into seeking to have another family member named the legal guardian, and taking all financial and legal rights away from the older person. This scenario happens mostly in cases involving an older person suffering with advanced dementia. Families should tread carefully in these situations; they don't want to initiate a meltdown or a family fight. No one wins when the older individual is not agreeable to the planned changes, and views any attempt to reduce their autonomy as an attack on them, personally. Once a previously beloved family member or friend is recast as the adversary, it becomes almost impossible to reestablish the prior image of trust. Talking to a representative at the bank may reveal many techniques that others have used successfully in these situations: needing a double signature before the bank honors the check; having a separate checking account in a guardian's" name; taking some of the burden of paperwork out of the hands of the elderly relative; etc. Close family members know their relative the best, and can seek help about what options are available. They then can choose the one that they feel is best suited for their relative.

Driving is another factor that is important to today's elderly population. Driving a car is viewed as another symbol of independence, and being in control of one's environment. Any suggestion that an older person should no longer drive can initiate a fight. It has important psychological value, as well as practical importance. Difficulties with driving by the older impaired person stem from several issues commonly encountered. Development of cataracts frequently causes a glare in bright light. Driving at night with cataracts produces a glare from the oncoming car headlights or lights in the rearview mirror. Furthermore, less light reaches the retina (due to more opacity of the cataract), and night vision will be impaired. The individual will not be able to see things and obstacles as well in the dim nighttime light. Older people realize this when it happens, and usually give up night driving. Glaucoma, macular degeneration, and a decreasing visual field of processing attention all affect the driving safety of an older person. Families become concerned when an elderly relative stays too long at a party, and plans to drive home long after it gets dark. Secondly, reaction time slows, leading to a slower braking response when there is a sudden need to brake. Drifting while making left turns through the oncoming traffic can cause accidents. Neck stiffness can make the older person rely more on looking through the mirror (with its blind spots) than turning the head when backing up or making turns. Arthritis in the hips, feet, and shoulders can bring on acute and sharp pain with braking, turning the wheel, or changing gears. This pain can interfere with required rapid movements.

Becoming involved in fender-benders is a frequent reason for many elderly to abandon driving. Children sometimes become very concerned when their elderly parent is still driving alone, or chauffeuring their grandchildren about. They are then caught in a bind. They don't want to upset the older parent, nor get into a battle with them, but they worry about their parent's safety and the safety of anyone in the car with them (and everyone else on the road). Insurance companies usually raise the premiums of car insurance on their older customers. Taking a state DMV-approved accident-prevention driving class can lower these premiums. There are courses specifically designed for the older driver. These courses are excellent, and taking such a course can alert the older driver about any personal difficulties they may be experiencing without threatening them as a personal attack. The more-impaired older driver will probably not pass this exam.

Many diseases can lead to issues regarding driving capacity, and state departments of motor vehicles or DMVs have lists of disorders that must be reported. If in doubt about the capacity of an older person to drive, a practical solution is to recommend the individual go to a driving school, and have a driving instructor take them out on a road test. If they do well, everyone can rest a little easier; if they fail, any recommendations come from the driving instructor. Alternatively, one can also inquire whether the local DMV can take the older individual out on a free road test. If all else fails, and the impaired relative still insists on driving, I sometimes inform them that if they are ever in an accident, and their medical records are examined, the other party will probably successfully sue them for everything they and their family possess. They are risking the future financial welfare of their family by driving.

Having an elderly relative living alone commonly causes much apprehension and fear in the family. Are they safe? Are they eating? Who's looking after them? This is particularly a problem if the relative is living a great distance from the concerned family. Techniques that have been used include having a local case manager (CM) who oversees the status of the older person. The CM periodically makes home visits, checks out the refrigerator and pantry for presence of adequate food and supplies, sees how the individual looks, and judges how well the older person is managing. It's like having a trained second person being the family's surrogate on the ground. The case manager usually also arranges for doctor's visits, and can even accompany the older relative on the visit.

"Life-lines" (or alerts) are popular, and provide an older person living alone with a means to call for help in an emergency; all they need to do is push a button, and someone will respond. Having a button to push in an emergency that summons immediate aid is very reassuring to the family, and to the patient as well. Like an alarm company, there is a 24/7 service always there to respond to the life-line alert.

More and more choices of where to live have been imagined and created. In the past there was the individual's own home, or an "old-age home" or "nursing home." Today there are senior communities, assisted living, shared facilities, and new types of living arrangements springing up throughout the country. There are pros and cons to each choice. But the fact is that there now are many choices available. It's best to be aware of the benefits and differences between these living arrangements before an emergency situation develops. It's also best to discuss your preferences with your children and family, and visit the places you might be considering.

The Goal of Healthy Living

There are many books to be read, programs in which to participate, and health spas to patronize, all emphasizing "healthy living." We all have been indoctrinated with this concept of healthy living. But what is "healthy living?" What does it entail, and could, or should this be our primary goal for living? Should older people start "healthy living" even after having lived an "unhealthy life"? Would it do any good? Is "healthy living" even essential to being healthy?

Patients frequently admit they do not follow a healthy diet, nor live a healthy lifestyle. But, as mentioned several times already, the primary goal of life is not to live a "healthy life." People live the lives they enjoy —whether "healthy" or otherwise. They have made their choices (hopefully an informed choice). It is sad that they should feel a need to apologize for who they are. Living a lifestyle that they acknowledge is not healthy adds to their guilt and depression.

Being healthy is always preferred, as long as it doesn't carry the burden of giving up too many things the individual enjoys, or requires too much effort. Whatever process went into their lifestyle choices, the individual felt the advantages of that type of living outweighed the disadvantages, assuming they had a choice. Being healthy not only allows one to enjoy life more, but also reduces the burden on family members who would have to care for the ill relative. From my perspective, healthy living means considering the health benefits associated with the choices we make.

It is healthy for the mind and body to be active. After retirement, it is important to fill the time vacuum with activities that give pleasure and satisfaction. Those older people who seem to be aging well have found renewed or new interests in volunteering, traveling, gardening, photography, reading, music, painting and sculpture, or taking courses in subjects they never previously had enough time to enjoy. They reinvent themselves with new projects and challenges. Throughout life, the mind should be kept active with learning. The list of things that can fill this list is endless. With retirement there should finally be time to indulge in all the activities for which there previously was "never enough time." It is always best to retire *to* something rather than *from* something. Each person judges what kind of life he or she wishes to live. Food should be enjoyed, and activities should be chosen by the degree of pleasure they impart. An intelligent person balances the pros and cons in anything they do.

Sexual activity and sexual drives do not end with the acquisition of gray hair. Frequently older people inquire about the safety of having sex. There is a strain on the heart with sexual intercourse, and people who have had previous heart attacks, or angina pectoris, are rightly concerned about safety issues. The current wisdom is that despite any underlying heart or lung disease, if a person can climb two flights of stairs without difficulty, they are healthy enough to engage in sex. Although there are hormonal changes (in women with menopause), and men with diminished testosterone activity (a kind of andropause), a normal and healthy life includes sexual activities. In both men and women, sexual interest is related to testosterone activity in the brain and can continue throughout their lives. (Women make testosterone by converting estrogens into testosterone.)

Depression, as well as taking many different types of medicines for high blood pressure and heart disease, can reduce sexual libido and cause impotence; some medications actually increase sexual libido. Neuropathies (discussed above), caused by diabetes, thyroid disease, etc., can lead to male impotence (nerves control blood flow to the penis, which causes the erection). Prostate cancer and some of its older surgical and nonsurgical treatments regularly led to male impotence. Medicines, used to shrink the prostate in men with prostatic hypertrophy, work by reducing the production of dihydrotestosterone (DHT), the most active form of testosterone. This can reduce libido. After menopause, women will experience drying of the vaginal lining, making intercourse more painful, and making lubricants more essential. In both sexes, more time is needed for sexual arousal. Many older men are now asking for medicines to combat "erectile dysfunction." The massive advertising campaign seen on TV has had its intended result. Pharmaceutical companies that manufacture these drugs know that older people can still enjoy sexual activity. The old adage "Use it, or lose it" is as applicable to sexual activity as it is to so many other things in life.

Having healthy teeth is important for good living—and good eating. The bones that anchor the teeth in the mouth are the mandible (the jaw bone), and maxilla (on top). These bones also age and undergo osteoporosis. As the bone reabsorbs and shrinks, teeth become less well anchored, and can loosen. Infections in the gum occur, and the gum itself shrinks, leaving more of the tooth exposed. This results in more tooth decay and greater loosening of teeth until they fall out. Enamel can be worn off. The addition of fluoride to municipal drinking water (something that was not performed in years past, when older people were young) has reduced the number of people today needing full dentures. Those who drink bottled water, or water from a well, should discuss fluoride treatments with their dentist. The bones in the mouth also require stress and exercise to maintain their strength, and if they are not stressed in chewing, they loosen and decay more.

With poor dental function, the individual becomes limited in what they can eat and enjoy, reducing the quality of their lives. Aside from pain and discomfort in the mouth, infections in the mouth can lead to infections elsewhere, such as pneumonia, abscesses, and infections of the bones of the mouth. Good dental prophylactic care is important in maintaining general good health. However, dental procedures, even dental examinations, performed on demented patients pose significant problems. Cooperation with the dentist will probably be lacking. Anesthesia and hospitalization may be needed.

There is good evidence that exercise is helpful for the circulation, the heart, the bones, the lungs, and the muscles. For exercise, some people just walk, others join a gym to exercise, and others hire a trainer. Some older people add stretching exercises or yoga. These are very good practices to keep joints limber. The important thing is to do something. By getting off an elevator one floor lower and climbing one flight of stairs, or parking at the far end of a parking lot and walking farther, or getting off a bus or subway one exit earlier and walking more, a person can add a considerable amount of additional exercise to their weekly activity. Exercise and physical activity has been repeatedly shown to be helpful for one's health. There is a difference between exercise and physical or occupational therapy. Physical therapy requires a trained therapist (not a trainer). The therapist directs the individual into doing some activity that is intended to improve a specific condition.

Similarly, a good diet has been shown to be helpful for health. Restriction of fats, salt, and "empty calories" is appropriate. But taste and smell are two of our five senses, and pleasurable eating and drinking adds much value to one's quality of life. Perhaps the old adage "all things in moderation" is a good mantra. As indicated above, fluids are an essential component of the diet, and the one component that is usually the most deficient in the elderly. We currently believe it is good to have some fiber in our diet. Vitamin and mineral supplements may be valuable in people with restricted diets. There are well documented vitamin deficiency states, which require the supplementation of vitamins that should normally have been in their food and diet: vitamin D, B12, folic acid, B complex, vitamin C, co-enzyme Q-10, Omega 3, vitamin E, as examples. There is good data to support their added intake in *some, but not all* individuals. For other supplements, the evidence is shaky. Glucosamine helps many with arthritis, but this supplement contains glucose. The reader should understand that the health supplement business is a multi-million-dollar industry that is trying to promote their products for their own profit. There is nothing wrong with this, but consumers should look to these supplements and health products with the same skepticism they would with any other product being heavily promoted by an aggressive salesman. Many older people, who may in fact need them, rarely take these supplements. Some older people use complete dietary formulas as caloric supplements to what they eat. The consumption of these "complete" liquid supplements in people who are able eat regular food is increasing dramatically, and for many reasons. For some, chewing and swallowing is difficult and the supplement goes down better. In others, the supplements offer a cheaper and easier way to get nutrition than would be obtained by purchasing, cooking, and eating regular food. In still others with financial problems, supplements can be obtained through their medical drug plan at no, or minimal, expense to them—it's free food.

Many of us grew up with the image of a food pyramid, which stressed that we needed daily consumption of five food groups for a healthy diet: dairy, meat, grain, fat, and vegetables. We were strongly advised to include elements of each of these groups daily. But humans have a great capacity to adapt to their diet. The traditional Inuit diet has no fruit, vegetables, or grains, but people survived in the Arctic climate in apparent reasonably good health. Natives of the Kalahari Desert in Africa live mostly on grains. People choose to become vegan, or vegetarian, limiting their diet, yet they seem healthy. Having a variety of foods to eat seems to fill the need to consume all of the essential vitamins. Severely restricted diets are associated with nutritional deficiencies. The truth is that humans, as a species, survived on this planet for hundreds of thousands of years without taking additional vitamins and supplements. They survived by eating and drinking what was there in their environment. Obviously those that could not adapt did not survive. We are the descendants of only those who could adapt, and who survived long enough to procreate. We are adapters.

Are the food supplements and "energy bars and drinks" helpful or necessary? People have their own ideas of what they believe is appropriate and healthy for them. The question for the physician is whether their diet and activities are harmful. If the doctor believes a person's diet is not healthy, the doctor should discuss this with the patient. However, if the person appears healthy and energetic, there is no need to change or advise anything.

A healthy life also implies trying to avoid infections. We are born with a variety of natural defenses. These defenses, however, do also age. The immune system ages with time, and diminished host defenses leave older people more vulnerable to many types of infections. Prevention of infection is always better than treatment. Four immunizations are currently recommended for all older people: (1) Influenza: This is an annual vaccination, as each year the recommended vaccine changes to include those strains of influenza that are anticipated by the experts to be problem strains capable of producing excessive disease in our susceptible community. Although forty thousand Americans die each year from seasonal flu (statistically the largest "preventable" disease), only two-thirds of people who should be immunized are immunized. (2) Pneumococcal, or "pneumonia":. The pneumococcus is a type of bacteria that can cause pneumonia, meningitis, and blood disseminated infections. It is not strictly a pneumonia vaccine, and does not protect against pneumonias caused by other germs. Although new vaccines for pneumococci are being offered, the most widely available vaccine for adults contains materials from twenty-three of the over one hundred types of pneumococcus that are responsible for the most common and serious infections. The pneumococcus is still the most common bacteria causing community pneumonia. (3) Tetanus toxoid: Tetanus is no longer a disease of children (who are almost all sufficiently immunized), but is now a disease of the elderly, whose skin is more fragile and easily disrupted by falls, burns, abrasions, cuts, etc. One doesn't need a rusty nail to get tetanus—any break in the skin can open a portal for the tetanus spores to enter. The immunization is effective, and should be given every ten years. We now are recommending the tetanus toxoid be given with diphtheria and pertussis (whooping cough) toxoid. A "toxoid" is a toxin that has been altered to eliminate the toxic nature of the poison, but maintains the immunological aspects of the parent molecule. (4) Shingles vaccine (Zostavax): Shingles develops only in people who have had chicken pox, and whose immunity has since waned below a critical threshold value. This attenuated live virus vaccine is now recommended for everyone over sixty years of age (and approved for everyone over fifty) as a one-time immunization, even if a person had had shingles previously. The inherent problem with immunization of the most elderly in our society is that the very people in whom we are trying to boost immune responses are those who will have the poorest immune responses. But any added immunity is better than none. The diminished immunity in the elderly has one positive, beneficial feature—a decrease in allergic reactions in the very old.

Preventing an infection is also the purpose of individuals taking antibiotics before undergoing colonoscopies or major dental cleaning and manipulation. The rectum/colon and mouth are the parts of the body that are the most heavily coated (or colonized) with bacteria of various sorts (normally the types of germs in these two locations are very different from one another). If, during mouth or colon/rectal manipulation, bleeding should occur, it can be expected that germs can enter our inner tissues. It is a two-way opening: if blood can come out—germs can go in. We frequently see some mouth bleeding after vigorous dental brushing, or blood on the toilet paper after going to the bathroom. So why didn't we get sick? The truth is that our best defenses to bacterial invasion are in these locations. But with aging, and more aggressive dental and colon irritation, we press our luck, since some people do develop serious infections in their mouth or around their rectum after these procedures. Antibiotic prophylaxis is recommended for all individuals who had recent joint replacements (we don't want these artificial joints getting infected) or those with significant valvular heart disease before having any significant procedure in the mouth, colon, or toes, where significant bleeding can occur or is expected. The choice of antibiotic depends upon the location of likely irritation and the germs that normally reside there.

Humans are social creatures, and it is healthy to have social contacts throughout our lives. With aging, there may be fewer social interactions. Pet therapy has been shown to be very helpful for many older people who live alone. A dog is a good companion, and brings the added benefit of requiring the owner to exercise daily when taking the dog for a walk. Caring for a dog can therefore have a double benefit. A cat can also be a good companion, and doesn't require cleaning up in the street the way a dog does. But cats are less obedient, and can transmit more diseases with scratches and bites than dogs. Plant therapy can be valuable, as older people living alone have lots of "free time" and may enjoy horticulture and watching plants grow.

Hobbies and new activities can also bring in some extra cash that can be very helpful and can stimulate the mind and exercise the body. Quilting, painting, photography, and jewelry-making are all activities that can produce added income while keeping the older person active, stimulated, and intellectually challenged. Innovative older people can certainly use their "extra time" for activities that keep them busy and are emotionally rewarding and financially helpful.

SECTION III — BEING AN OLDER PATIENT

As for old age, embrace and love it. It abounds with pleasure if you know how to use it. The gradually declining years are among the sweetest in a man's life, and I maintain that, even when they have reached the extreme limit, they have their pleasure still.

SENECA

Being an informed patient, and being an effective partner with your doctor and health team, requires some understanding of what being a patient is all about. It might be useful to keep in mind that the whole health-care system, with all its complex components, exists to take care of the patient. Patients don't exist to take care of the system. The patient is the central core component. Don't be intimidated. This section deals with the delivery of health care.

Reducing Confusion Taking Medications

The older population is the principal consumer of medications in our society. As the picture on the cover of this book suggests, some older people take many, many medications daily. Errors in taking medicine are more common in the elderly, and most can be avoided.

Some simple and avoidable mistakes are commonly made. Labels can be confusing, particularly if generics are substituted for brand names. If this happens, place a colored tag onto the medicine bottle and write the other name. If taking 2 different strengths of the same medicine (often the case with warfarin [Coumadin] or thyroid), contained in two separate bottles, put different color tags on each. Although it may be easier to carry, try not to put different medications into the same pill bottle (the problem of loose unlabeled pills leads to many errors). If you forget, or miss taking a particular medicine one day, don't panic, nor try to "double up" the next day to compensate for the day missed. Understand if any of the medicines you are taking are diet-dependent (e.g., warfarin, diabetic medicines, antihypertensives). With these medicines in particular, not eating, or changing the amount of vitamin K, sugar/carbohydrate, or salt, respectively, that you are consuming can influence the amount of medicine needed for proper control of your condition. Don't run out of a medicine and wait till the next doctor's appointment before asking for more. If running low, call the pharmacy or doctor for more refills. And, if your doctor had given you free samples of a medicine to "try," or had prescribed a small amount of the medicine to "see its effect," make sure you still are taking that medicine when you see your doctor next. If that medicine is out of your system at the time of your next examination, it will be impossible to determine its full effect (benefit or harm).

Medicines are expensive and seem to be getting more expensive; saving on medications can be a priority. Many people now search the Internet for cheaper medicines (usually coming from, or made, abroad). Others pick up medications during foreign travel, or ask contacts abroad to send them the cheaper products. We do hear of fake medicines entering the US market that are made abroad, and most of us are afraid to try these "cheaper" products as a result.

As discussed below, medications fall into various categories based on their mode of action. Insurance drug plans (discussed below) vary greatly in which medications they prefer their covered clients to use—based solely on the cost. A good deal of money can be saved by asking the prescribing physician whether there is a specific need for a particular medication, or whether another medicine in the same category (that is cheaper), can be tried first. Most often, it is the *effect* or activity of the drug that is important, and if that effect is accomplished with a cheaper drug—so much the better. The insurance company, under which the person has their drug coverage, or the pharmacist can advise the patient as to whether there is a cheaper alternative medicine that is covered under the individual's chosen drug plan.

Errors in taking medicines fall into several types: taking the wrong medicine (or not taking it), taking the wrong dosage of medicine, taking the medicine at the wrong schedule, with the wrong foods, or with interfering medicines. In general, as a person ages and their metabolism slows, doses of medicines that were appropriate for a younger person can become too much for the older patient.

Improper management of medications represents a particular problem with the elderly. With the high cost of medicines and the considerable effort often needed to visit their doctor, many elderly try to maintain their own mini-pharmacies at home, tucked away in their medicine cabinet. There, they may have unused medicines of various sorts (many of which may be outdated), and there they like to keep antibiotics available, in case they get sick. Some also share these "stored," unused medicines with their friends and neighbors.

The individual may perceive a benefit in having a pharmacy of needed medicines at home and easily available, but may not realize the risk and penalty they take when they become their own prescriber. Some individuals also believe that, "if a little amount of the medicine helped a little, a lot more of the medicine should help a lot more." This philosophy doesn't work any better with medicines than it does in cooking. Stick to the prescribed instructions. Although ill elderly individuals may think it all right to try their own remedy first, they may delay having a proper diagnosis made, and can confound the clinical situation, making their later care more difficult.

Indiscriminant use of antibiotics is a major cause of developing antibiotic-resistant bacteria in the patient and in the community, and makes treating these resistant bacteria a major problem. This has become a major health hazard in our society. There is no antibiotic to which all germs are sensitive. Taking the wrong antibiotic for the wrong diagnosis can be harmful to the individual, causing unnecessary fungal and severe intestinal infections.

Flushing unused or outdated medicines down the toilet is another no-no. Many medicines, including antibiotics and hormones, end up in streams or waters where there are living fish or plants, and can affect our entire biosphere. Prescription medicines are entering our food chain, and are becoming an increasing public health problem. Many communities collect old medicines, as they do old computers and toxic wastes, for more appropriate disposal. Old, unused medicines around the house should be stored in a closed container (an old jar, milk, or juice container) until time for collection and disposal by proper means.

Then there is the problem of older people opening pill bottles. Unless specifically instructed otherwise, the pharmacist will most likely dispense medicines in a "childproof" bottle that is extremely difficult for most elderly to open. The consequence of this protective cap is that many elderly do not close the lids of their medicine bottles securely, and pills spill out—everywhere. When coming to the office, there is a routine of opening the zip-lock bag in which they brought their medicines, and trying to match each loose pill with the bottle and label from which they originally came. There often are loose tablets and capsules in pockets or loose in handbags. Older patients should ask the pharmacist if the medicines could be dispensed in a more easily opened container. This will avoid a lot of frustration, the risk of taking the wrong medicine (taking a medicine based on its appearance, not its name), and knife injuries sustained while trying to open pill bottles.

There is also a significant risk of "polypharmacy"—taking an awful lot of different medications, and running the risk of adverse drug interactions. The more medicines a person takes, the greater the risk of drug interactions, drugs that interfere with one another, and drug noncompliance.

Many patients take their medications regularly, and as prescribed, but intentionally refrain from taking them on the day of the doctor's appointment. Taking a diuretic on the day when traveling to the doctor, in a not too toilet-friendly environment, can lead to an embarrassing situation. Further, taking the extra fluid needed to swallow their pills that morning may also lead to problems. They also often hold off on taking their medicines on this day due to an erroneous belief that their doctor may want to do blood tests, and taking the medicines that day would interfere with the testing. When queried about taking their medicines, they respond that they are taking them daily, but somehow omit to mention that they did NOT take them on the day of the visit. The doctor may then mistakenly think the medicine is not working, as when the blood pressure is still high after prescribing a blood-pressure medicine. There is a good possibility that the medicines will then be increased, and the patient asked to return to evaluate the response. If the patient again does not take the medicine on the day of the visit, the patient runs the risk of the doctor raising the dosage of medicines still again, etc. A variant of this problem occurs when a doctor is trying out a new medicine and prescribes a limited number of pills to last till the next appointment, when their benefit can be determined. If not enough pills are given, or the patient postpones the appointment, it is not uncommon for the patient to come for the appointment having finished this "trial" medicine several days earlier. It is then impossible to know if the medication had any benefit on the blood pressure, heart rate, breathing, etc., because its effect would no longer be observable. The patient should inform the doctor if she had *not* taken the medicines that day; and doctors should ask that critical question.

Each medication has three names: a chemical name, a brand name, and a generic name. The public is often confused about the latter two. It is not by accident that generic names are difficult to pronounce and are generally three to four syllables long, whereas brand names are easier to remember and may be only one or two syllables. When a pharmaceutical company releases a new product, after receiving FDA permission, only the brand name product is initially available in pharmacies. The company normally has eight to ten years to market their product without any generic competition[3].

---

3 The process of getting a new medicine to market generally takes eight to twelve years. A patent for most new drugs is for twenty years. A brand-name medicine therefore has between eight and twelve years before any competitive generics become available.

After this time, anyone who wishes can make the product and sell it under the generic name, provided they get approval from the FDA, which still must approve its efficacy and safety. A generic medication is neither required to be the same color nor the same shape as the comparable brand name. There also may be several generics competing for the same market, each with their own appearance. These differences often cause confusion in the public. With a "refill" of their prescription, they notice a different name on the bottle (often unpronounceable), and may even find a different-appearing medicine. They may be afraid to take the "new" pill, believing a mistake was made. If there is a question about the medicine being dispensed, they should consult the pharmacist.

Since generic drugs are usually cheaper than the brand name, insurance companies that pay for medications generally encourage the consumer to use the generic whenever possible. On most prescriptions, only if the prescribing individual marks "daw" (dispense as written), or specifically asks for the brand name, will the brand name be dispensed. Even then, the insurance company may ask for justification in why a more expensive brand-name medicine is being prescribed. For most medications, the generic medicine is just as good as the brand name product.

The FDA monitors the quality and potency of the generic. The FDA also requires that the generic be comparable in strength and activity to the brand, but there can be differences. Generics can be 10–15 percent more or less active than the brand, which usually does not make too much of a difference.

It is important to realize that in addition to the active medicine ingredient, medications contain "inert" materials such as fillers, binders, coloring agents, and preservatives. Sometimes individuals develop allergies and reactions to these "inert" ingredients that may be unique to that preparation, but blame the intolerance on the active ingredient—the big name on the label.

They then carry this "allergic" label with them for the rest of their life.

It is very important that patients learn the names of the medicines they take. This is not easy, because the names may not be familiar and generic names are particularly hard to pronounce. It is worth the time and effort to learn and practice pronouncing the names, and remembering the strengths of every medicine being taken. If a doctor asks the patient what medicines they are taking, and gets a blank stare, it looks bad for the patient, and can take the doctor an extra ten to fifteen minutes trying to call the pharmacy or a relative who might know what medications the person is taking. These are important pieces of information.

As a safety backup, or if remembering all the medications is too difficult, patients should also maintain an updated list of medications that they take, including the dosage and times of day they take each of their medicines. They should keep this list on their person and in a convenient place in their home near the medications. If ever the emegency medical service (EMS) needs to visit the person, they are trained to bring all the medications in the medicine cabinet with the patient as they take them to the hospital or emergency room. The emergency room (ER) staff use these medicines and the labeled instructions as indicators of what the patient is actually taking, and try to continue all the essential meds. Sometimes this leads to problems, if those medicine-cabinet bottles are mislabeled or incomplete. Old, or medications no longer used, should not be kept with active currently used medications. If the individuals have reduced the dose by cutting the pills in half (a cost-saving measure many people practice), this should be so indicated on the label.

Some medications are very dependent upon diet. Warfarin, or Coumadin, a medicine to slow blood clotting, is very dependent upon the amount of vitamin K in the diet. The dose prescribed is carefully adjusted according to the person's particular sensitivity to the medicine, aiming for a target effect. If, for whatever reason, an individual taking warfarin loses their appetite, or is not eating, the vitamin K in the diet can drop to zero, and the effect of the warfarin is now unopposed; the anticlotting effect can be excessive and the person can bleed badly. They may not be aware of the increased risk of bleeding nor of any slow bleeding initially, unless they are actively hemorrhaging, and will not likely seek medical attention until they notice they are vomiting blood, feel weak, faint, and sweaty, or see blood in their urine or feces.

Diabetic medicines are similarly dependent upon the diet. If an individual is not eating, taking the "normal" amount of insulin or other diabetes medicines can produce a severe drop in blood sugar. This will produce symptoms of sweating, lightheadedness, nausea, or even passing out. Antihypertensive medications are also adjusted to a particular person's need, and if that person changes the amount of salt in their diet, the medications will need adjustment. This may, or may not, produce new symptoms of headache or malaise (if the pressure is too high), or a sense of passing out (if the pressure is too low). With any of these types of medicines, a change in appetite or diet should signal a warning alarm to check in with their prescribing physician. Losing or gaining weight can also affect how much medicine will be needed to control blood pressure or diabetes.

Changes in medicines also happen when people are admitted to a hospital. Unlike a community pharmacy, the hospital pharmacy does not carry all the medications that individuals might be taking at home. They will stock representative medications of important pharmaceutical groups. By limiting which medications of any particular class or purpose they will carry, they can negotiate prices with their distributors in a way much more to their advantage. This too leads to some patient confusion. When they are admitted to the hospital, patients may be prescribed alternate medications that have the same effect as the ones they took at home, but have different names. The doses of many of these medications may be different, because of different efficacy of the medicines, and also because the diet and stresses encountered in the hospital are different from those encountered at home. After discharge, the individual may need (with the aid of their physician) to readjust their medications back to what they took before hospitalization.

Taking medications at home as prescribed can be another problem. Which medications should be taken with food? Which without any other medicines? Which in the morning, and which at night? Older persons are taking, on the average, at least three different prescribed medicines and one to two over-the-counter medicines daily. (These over-the-counter medications are also pharmaceuticals, and should be included in the patient's own drug list.) Some of my patients take fifteen to twenty different medications daily. When the medication instructions become too complicated (one medicine prescribed as every eight hours; another twice a day; another before or after meals and another before "bedtime"), it is almost impossible to take the medicines as directed and mistakes will be made. This problem is compounded when a person is seeing several physicians. Each physician prescribes medicines independently; taking into account what other medications the patient is taking (thus avoiding possible adverse drug interactions), but not taking into account the time schedules for taking these medicines. Taking medicines as directed can become the main focus of the day, and the individual can spend their entire day looking at the clock, and taking their medicines as told. That is not what living is supposed to be. Many people just take the medicines at their convenience, disregarding the actual directions. For some disorders, like Parkinson's disease, the timing can be critical. I recommend that when the regimen becomes too complicated, the patient talk to the prescribing individual, or their primary doctor about simplifying the drug schedule and if all the medicines are really necessary. Compromises may have to be made. Most doctors are unfamiliar with the cost of the various medications (just as the patients are not familiar with the price until handed a bill at the pharmacy). Patients should not be embarrassed about asking whether there are cheaper versions of the medications that might have the same effect. (See discussion below about Medicare part D—drug plan insurance).

Pharmacies and Internet sites list all the potential problems that have been reported in people taking the medication. The FDA demands the listing of all adverse reactions that have been observed if they occur more frequently than 1–3 percent of the time (but this also means it doesn't happen 97 percent of the time). Some of these "adverse" reactions are clearly due to the medication; sometimes they are only minimally more frequent than that observed when people were taking placebo. Sometimes the link or causality of the adverse reaction to the medicine is not clear. "Someone took a pill, and then fell down." Nonetheless, for legal purposes, and to forewarn the consumer, these potential reactions are publicized.

An individual who reads these theoretical risks and worries about the safety of the medication will probably be afraid to take any medicine; they should discuss their actual risk with the doctor. Many times the patient senses that he or she has all the symptoms and complaints listed as possible problems associated with his or her medicines. How do you determine whether a medicine is hurting, or helping? Obviously, you should discuss this with your doctor, who can then draft a plan of slow elimination of a drug for its effect, shift the time of administration of the medicine, or eliminate those medicines that can be stopped abruptly. Many medicines cannot be stopped abruptly, but need slow weaning. This point should be emphasized. Never stop a medicine abruptly unless your doctor says this can be done safely. If your doctor did not mention how to stop the medicine, it pays to ask.

Making changes in the prescribed medicines without supervision is very dangerous. Often, the risk of not taking a needed medicine vastly outweighs the risk of taking the medicine. Once again there develops the need to judge the benefit-to-risk ratio. Taking over-the-counter medicines also has potential risks, as does taking nonproprietary supplements and vitamins. Very little in life is totally risk-free. I often need to remind a patient that just because something is "natural" does not mean that it's safe. There are a lot of "natural" poisons out there.

Some older patients readily accept the recommendations, advice, and medications being proffered by their friends and neighbors above that of their doctor. It is that they know and trust their friends and neighbors more than they do a new doctor (who they may not "be sure of yet"). When a friend tells them that they improved with a different medicine than the one given by their doctor, they are drawn to trying it. This can obviously be very frustrating for the doctor.

The actual management of an older person's medications can become a complicated undertaking. Organization is the key. There are pillboxes, pill organizers, and electronic pill reminders, that can be set up by the day, the week, or several weeks. Some pharmacies remind patients that a refill of their medication is due. It is helpful to go over one's medications with the doctor at each visit. Sometimes patients are still taking medications that the doctor believes were discontinued long ago; other times new prescriptions were never filled.

Making Sense of Test Results

Laboratory tests are best used when selectively ordered to assist in making the diagnosis. They may contribute 20 percent of the information employed in making a final diagnosis when used appropriately in the proper situation. They should not be used as a broad fishing net blindly cast out to see what shows up. As discussed below, inappropriate testing will not be paid for by the insurance company, and can be very expensive for the patient, if the individual is asked to pay himself.

Many patients seem to be overly focused on the results of their laboratory tests. They become very disturbed when they see a value that is flagged as being high or low. To understand this better, a little understanding of the statistical terms *normal variation* and *normal distribution* is important. We are not all alike. Results of healthy people will not be identical. The laboratory highlights a deviation from normal if a result is 5 percent off from the average, expected value. When 20 independent tests are done, just by statistical variation, one value will likely be statistically "abnormal" in a normal person. Furthermore, there is variation in results with duplicate testing. With some tests, the same study is done in duplicate (as with calcium measured both in concert with the hormone, parathyroid hormone, and as part of the normal battery of tests). The bloods were taken at the same time, but the tests were done separately, and the results are rarely identical. If bloods were taken every hour from an individual, or ten duplicate tests were made with the same blood sample, you would quickly see that there is a range of results that reflect the variability between the assays. Instead of focusing on the absolute number, try to think of results as "OK," "too low," or "too high."

Secondly, the absolute value of a test result is not nearly as important as the trend of results. It is in the context of the complaints, and how it has changed over time, that there is meaning. A perspective is needed. An abnormal laboratory test that is improving or is stable is reassuring. An X-ray that shows a "shadow" (something absorbing the X-rays) is of some concern, but when the image has not changed over many years, it is of little significance in an asymptomatic patient. Looking at an isolated test result only causes stress and anxiety when it is flagged as "abnormal."

Lastly, many patients request the frequent examination of their laboratory test results, and ask that copies of all test results be sent to them. Perhaps some of this attitude and focus on test results originates from doctors who place great emphasis on laboratory tests. When hospitalized, patients often are subjected to repetitive testing of their blood on a daily basis (and sometimes multiple times a day), as ordered by an intern (PGY-1, see below) or junior physician (this is particularly true in teaching hospitals where medical orders are frequently written by the house staff). At times the test results are truly needed; but sometimes they are obtained for "defensive" reasons (medico-legal fears), because of young doctor insecurity, because of a questionably needed protocol, or because the orders, which had been written at an earlier time when there was greater diagnostic uncertainty, had not been cancelled. A psychological consequence of this repeated testing in the hospital is the risk that the patient will develop a false impression about the need for testing. Another consequence of testing frequently is the cost in money, blood, and utilization of time and materials needed for testing. Patients should protect their blood, and question the doctor (in the hospital or in the office) about whether all the tests are *really* necessary at that frequency.

It is not necessary to measure the cholesterol every one to three months; just as it is not necessary to repeat the PSA, vitamin D, and many other laboratory tests with each visit. This repeated testing is unnecessary, and just feeds into the mistake of treating laboratory values ahead of the patient. Some people have a fascination, even an obsession, about test results, constantly worrying about some undiscovered abnormality. Excessive testing feeds into this behavior by focusing attention on laboratory results (doctors should be trying to treat patients and their problems, not laboratory results). Laboratory testing is a supplemental aid to diagnosis. The major tools in making a diagnosis are still the patient's history and the physical examination. Excessive testing adds tremendously to the cost of health care. The average battery of laboratory tests costs hundreds of dollars. The doctor can be asked when the last examination of the particular blood test was done, but should not be pressured into repeating it unnecessarily.

Insurance companies sometimes limit the places where medical testing can be done. In general, patients should realize that there are two types of tests. Standard laboratory tests of blood and urine are done by machines, which are pretty much the same the world over. The results are standardized, usually reproducible, and would be the same regardless of where the test was done. In these tests, therefore, there is no problem in doing these studies at the most convenient laboratory that meets the patient's needs. The other type of test involves a strong professional component, and the results are not standardized. These include taking and interpreting X-rays, ultrasounds, echocardiograms, nuclear studies, etc. In these studies, not only is a good image important, but also your treating doctor relies strongly on the opinion of the person interpreting the result. As a consequence, the doctor may request that the study be done at a particular location and interpreted by a person or persons in whom the doctor has confidence. One should not just go to anyplace where there is a machine.

Aside from laboratory test results, even results of the physical examination can be misunderstood. Invariably, patients complain about their weight as measured on the physician's scale. It is never as low as their weight at home. People generally want to weigh less, and are disturbed when they see their weight in the doctor's office. At home, weights are generally measured early in the morning after going to the bathroom. This is a base weight, with an empty bladder, an empty colon, and an empty stomach, with no edema fluid yet collected in the legs, and with the individual naked. The weight in the doctor's office is used only as a reference (and it's confidential). It is the change in weight that is of clinical importance, not the absolute accuracy of the measured weight. Measured weight can be affected by clothes, and how long it's been since the person last went to the bathroom.

Similarly, people get disturbed about their blood pressure. One should recognize that the "vital signs" of blood pressure, heart rate, and breathing rate are not fixed rates, but dynamic values, influenced by activity, diet, and stress. It was a survival advantage to be able to adapt to stress in our environment. What would it mean if you were breathing rapidly, your heart was pounding fast, and your blood pressure was high if you were rushing to an appointment to which you were already late? It would be a very different meaning if those high rates were found while you were sleeping or relaxing on a beach. This is why these measurements need to be taken several times during rest, and interpreted in the context of what was happening in the person's life. The blood pressure is an important number, and some older people need a greater pressure for adequate circulation. If, on examination, there is evidence of damage in the eyes, kidneys, heart, and blood vessels caused by the high blood pressure, then there is no question that lowering the pressure is a priority. Blood pressure is also affected by sodium (salt) intake, and by stress (internal or external). A person can expect his blood pressure to be higher the day after ingesting a large, salty meal (e.g., marinara sauce, sushi with soy sauce, or pastrami). Similarly, if they are stressed by the very act of having their pressure taken, the pressure can be increased (this is the so-called white coat syndrome). Measured blood pressure is altered by changes in heart rate or rhythm (see p. 80). Some individuals buy their own blood pressure device (a sphygmomanometer), or wear a twenty-four-hour blood pressure recording device (about which there is now increasing doubt of reliability). We are made to tolerate short periods of higher pressure, but should not be subjecting our hearts and blood vessels to prolonged excessive pressure. It is the calculus of how high, and for how long, the pressure was elevated that deserves attention.

When women have had breast cancer, they are told not to let anyone take blood or measure blood pressure from the arm of the affected side. The reason for this is that the lymph nodes in the corresponding armpit may have been removed or affected by radiation or surgery. If, with the surgery, any scarring has occurred, it is possible that the arteries have become pinched, and the pressure on that side would be less a reliable indicator of the real blood pressure. Also, as a result of treating the breast cancer, there may be more swelling or edema on that side (which can interfere with measurement of the blood pressure by all the insulating effect of the lymphedema). And, lastly, if there were to be any irritation or infection from taking blood from the arm, or from the trauma of measuring the blood pressure, it is better to use the unaffected arm. This proscription should be a guide, not an absolute rule. When women have bilateral breast cancer or mastectomies, they panic about where blood will be removed, and how a blood pressure can be measured.

Trying to Figure Out Your Health Insurance Coverage

Dealing with your health insurance company risks losing your composure, if not your sanity. Health-insurance coverage is a world unto itself, and, at least in the United States, is very, very complicated. Most Americans, of any age, are unclear about what medical coverage they actually have, and only learn what is and what is not covered when they try to collect reimbursement for their medical bills and the money they had laid out. They may have to fight in order to get approval or reimbursement for their medical care.

After receiving medical care, particularly after a hospitalization during which a procedure was performed, you will receive bills, and many of them: bills from every professional, service, and department involved in your care (see section below on coding and billing). Suffice it to say, you may be shocked by the number of bills generated by the different services involved in your care. You will be involved in full-time correspondence with your health-insurance companies as well as your medical providers. Be prepared, and be organized. It may help to set up book-keeping sheets (or spreadsheets) with headings such as: date, service, original charge, date and amount insurance company paid, residual amounts, other insurance payments, and amounts you were responsible for paying.

Probably everyone has their own personal horror story about dealing with his or her health-insurance company. There are bills received from providers for services thought previously paid in full. Some patients may also receive checks from their health-insurance company that they know should have gone to their provider and they now have to deal with returning the money to the correct party. It is often a cause of great distress, confusion, and anger for both the patient and the provider (I'm not sure of how much of a distress it causes in the insurance company).

To resolve problems requires an enormous amount of patience, a good deal of luck, and connecting with the proper person who has the authority to correct the difficulty. Laws change, and company and insurance policies change. Each company has its own rules and regulations, and offers many different types and plans of insurance coverage (all for different premiums). Some companies covering a person's secondary insurance will send payment checks only to the provider, others only to the subscriber.

One should clarify what medical insurance one actually has before a new and particularly expensive type of care is planned. Providers and participants can and should inquire about an individual's specific coverage from the insurance company before the costs are incurred. A good rule to avoid later aggravation is, "When in doubt—ask!"—And, "When not in doubt—ask!"

The language that is used is the first thing that needs understanding: "covered expenses" and "noncovered expenses"; "participating" and "nonparticipating"; "accepting" and "nonaccepting"; "approved" and "nonapproved"; "full payment" and partial or residual payment; "primary" and "secondary" insurance, and deductibles. These categories can be mixed and matched for any particular service. A covered service performed by a nonparticipating provider who normally accepts assignment from the secondary insurance company, but not the primary, can lead to chaos.

Patients with Medicare as their primary health insurance have simpler issues. But Medicare rules and payments are also complex, and may change. The new Affordable Care Act (also known as "Obamacare") will no doubt, add another layer of confusion and uncertainty until its full provisions and requirements are fully implemented and are well understood by all parties. "Coordination of benefits" means that the involved insurance companies have worked out a plan in which they communicate between themselves for each company to pay its portion of the bill, without having the subscriber burdened with the task of determining proportional responsibilities and actual payments.

Some additional points need to be understood. Medicare Part A is automatic and free when a person becomes sixty-five; it pays 80 percent of approved hospital bills—0 percent for doctor's fees. It is generally for inpatient care. If a patient is in an institution for reasons that Medicare does not approve, Medicare can "carve out," or refuse to pay for these days. The patient may then be held financially responsible for those expenses (although the patient has to receive prior notification, and has a right to appeal this denial). There are also limits to the numbers of hospital days for which Medicare will pay: full pay for sixty days, then part pay for thirty days. There are also a finite number of "lifetime" days, *which are not renewable*, and after which Medicare will no longer pay. To "recharge" one's Medicare non-lifetime days (reset the full Medicare Part A coverage), a patient must be "out of the Medicare system"—i.e., no Medicare bills being generated by hospitals or institutions, for a period of sixty days.

Medicare Part B is optional, and must be purchased; it usually is taken out of a person's Social Security, and covers 80 percent of the medical provider's fees. There is an annual deductible for which the patient is responsible. The 80 percent begins only after the deductible amount has been met. Congress sets these provider fees each year, for each level of service, after the annual deductible has been met. The provider must have an approved provider number (i.e., be registered with Medicare). The individual is responsible for the annual deductible (currently $155) and the remaining 20 percent. (Note: Some physicians have dropped out of Medicare, no longer have an approved provider number, and their bill will not be paid by Medicare, leaving the full responsibility of payment to the patient –see p. 238). Medicare sets several fee schedules, depending upon whether the provider agrees to "participate" (this means accepting this fee as the total amount owed) and for which Medicare will send its share directly to the provider. There is a slightly higher fee schedule (usually 15 percent higher) for "nonparticipating" providers, who also must comply with Medicare's limiting rates.

Medicare-provider doctors can choose to "accept" or "not accept" assignment. If they choose not to accept, patients may have to pay the entire fee to the provider, and will be reimbursed by Medicare via a set fee reimbursement schedule (minus any annual deductible that remains). Providers who have "dropped out," or do not submit any bills to Medicare, can set any fee they want. Secondary insurance is the additional coverage a person buys from any one of a number of different private insurance companies that will cover the outstanding 20 percent of the Medicare reimbursement schedule, but also requires an annual deductible. These policies are very similar to each other, and not nearly as complicated as the private primary health-insurance policies described above.

There is also "Managed Medicare," or "Medicare Advantage" policies, or Medicare part C. In these policies, which are privately run, the insurance companies promise to cover all medical expenses, without any annual deductible, and with no additional fees being charged the patient. These policies are much cheaper than having the secondary insurance coverage for the 20 percent. So how can they afford to offer this kind of coverage? First of all, at the present time, they get a higher reimbursement from the government Medicare system than would be gotten from the traditional Medicare Part A and B. Secondly, they restrict access to care by allowing care to be given only by physicians, laboratories, therapists, or radiology services that agree to charge them a much lower fee than Medicare generally sets. Prior authorization is needed for any planned hospital admission, or approval is needed very soon after an emergency admission. Prior authorization is required for outpatient procedures such as colonoscopies, MRIs, or excision of skin lesions, as well as expensive inpatient procedures such as open-heart surgery. Prior authorization is needed for home antibiotics, nursing care, or therapy.

Because of lower payment rates and the burdens associated with getting prior approval and authorizations, many, if not most, physicians, laboratories, radiology services, etc., will not participate in these "managed" plans. This may make it difficult for the patient with Managed Medicare to get the services from the providers they want. For those with very limited income and high medical expenses, managed care plans should be seriously considered, as most have drug benefits and minimal, if any, co-pay. If the federal government reduces its generous payment to Medicare Advantage plans (as has been discussed), the conditions of these plans may change. It would also be prudent to investigate which doctors, clinics, or other anticipated providers in a person's community participate in the plan you are considering before you subscribe—and to read the fine print!

How are fee schedules determined? Generally, insurance companies annually determine their fee schedules based on the current fair and average market price of the services in any given community. The fee schedule in a high-rent urban center will be much higher than in a rural community. There have been challenges to the fairness of insurance fee schedules, claiming they used inaccurate data to their advantage. The subscriber rates they charge the consumer are based on their anticipated expenses and their need for profit.

If people are covered by an insurance policy from work, they may have that private insurance as their "primary" insurance, and may have a secondary insurance with Medicare or another private insurance company. Employers can switch health plans at any time, whenever they want, throwing the insured into a panic when they realize their new health insurance may have a different coverage policy than the plan they had previously been using—particularly if they are in the middle of some treatment procedure. Working spouses may have been assigned different health-insurance policies and plans from their employer, posing another layer of confusion. Most employer-provided health-insurance plans have "in-network" and "out-of-network" fee schedules. The "in-network" coverage is for providers who "participate" with that insurance company. "Out-of-network" may provide some payment for providers who are not participating with the insurance company, but generally covers only a part of the actual fee, if it covers anything at all. The participant must pay the full and regular fee of the "out-of-network" provider, and hope to receive partial reimbursement.

Medicaid or MediCal (the names change depending upon in which state the individual resides) is a state-run policy, and provides coverage for individuals who meet the income requirements of not being able to afford private medical insurance coverage. In patients who have Medicare as well, it picks up the 20 percent Medicare does not pay, as well as the annual deductible. These plans generally can provide for home attendants, all surgical supplies, medications, dental care, hearing aids, nursing home care, and generally all aspects of health care, including the annual deductible. These services are not covered under Medicare. Medicaid's reimbursement of the 20 percent to physicians is notoriously lower than 20 percent, and many physicians hesitate about accepting such patients into their practice. As another negative incentive, there is a constant need for various forms to be completed that burdens the provider. Medicaid reimbursement rates have been increasing, but current fiscal state matters may stop this trend.

Sometimes confusion arises as to which of two insurance companies is primary and which is secondary. This sometimes is the case when with a couple, each receives a different medical insurance from their employer, or a person gets medical insurance from multiple employers. In the coordination of benefits program, the insurance companies themselves will need to agree on which will be the primary and which the secondary insurance.

Medicare Part D is the nongovernment pharmaceutical coverage. This is a relatively new law that requires each person to have credible pharmaceutical insurance coverage. There are many insurance companies that sell such insurance at very different premiums. Each insurance company has its own list of which pharmaceuticals they will cover, how much the co-payments will be, the annual deductible, and how many pills they will allow with each prescription. Medications are assigned "tier" status (this is usually based on the cost of the medication, but the same medication can be assigned to different tiers by different companies). Tier One medications are generally generic, cheaper, and a ninety-day prescription will often be accepted. Tier Two medications are generally brand name, are more expensive, and have moderately high co-pay. How many pills will be dispensed with each prescription may vary with the policy. Tier Three medications are all brand name and expensive, and a much higher co-pay is required. Some medications need prior approval, and letters of necessity, explaining what other medications have been tried, and why this medication is necessary. Approval is not automatic, and often the medication requests are not granted. Some other medications are not covered at all. The insurance companies, at the present time, can change which medications they will pay for, and at which tier, anytime they want. The subscriber can only join or change their insurance company during the window beginning at the end of October to the end of the year. The law currently requires that the insurance company allow thirty-one days of medicines that have been removed from the company's formulary during the first ninety days of the patient's eligibility with the plan. The subscriber can also apply for an exemption to this policy. Patients with high drug costs can ask the pharmacist whether their out-of-pocket costs (with their particular insurance) would be cheaper with a different, but similarly active, medication. They can bring that information back to their prescribing physician and perhaps get a lower-tier substitute medicine.

In today's medical world, every insured individual has a unique patient identifier number that the insurance company recognizes and may assign. Every provider (physician, therapist, hospital, and practitioner) has his or her individual national provider number. Every test, procedure, level of care, therapy has its specific identifying number. And every diagnosis, for which testing or treatment is being ordered has its identifying number. All these various numbers (which are standardized across the country) must be supplied and are entered into the insurance company's computers. This allows the insurance company to track every aspect of an individual's health care for which they will need to pay. If the diagnosis code (called an ICD-9 code) does not justify the tests or procedures being ordered, the insurance company can refuse to pay. This can be very frustrating for patients, when told that the tests or procedures their doctor ordered are not covered because an inappropriate diagnosis code was entered. The providers are burdened with having to know which diagnoses the insurance company will accept and pay for, to justify the tests and procedures they want.

It is also important to recognize that health-insurance companies are there to make a profit. They prefer to have healthy patients who pay the premiums, but require little health care and minimal monetary expenditure. If a patient becomes a "high roller," needing expensive care, the insurance company would be delighted to have the patient change their coverage to another insurance company. To reduce their costs, the insurance companies may limit the subscriber to which laboratories, radiology services, or other services they can use. They prefer the patient go to places where they have negotiated lower fees. Patient convenience is not their top priority, although most insurance companies prefer to maintain a good image with their subscribers and with the community.

Long-term health insurance is another private insurance offered by many companies and usually targeted to the older population. The rather high premium increases as the party gets older and the reality of needing such coverage becomes a pressing issue. The insurance pays for home care and for nursing home care for a defined period, if the individual meets *their* corporate definition of being disabled and in need of such care. Many people as they age are attracted to this insurance, but hesitate in purchasing it because of its cost as well as the limited coverage.

If all of this discussion about health insurance is confusing, you are not alone. Individuals have great latitude in choosing just what kind of health insurance they wish, but the result of this abundance of options is that providers, as well as consumers, may not be clear about what exactly is covered and how much any procedure will cost them up front. In our health-insurance system, being an informed and wise consumer requires constant attention to details, vigilance, understanding the frequent changes in health plans, and stamina. These attributes are not usually present in an aging person, and the burden of dealing with health-insurance plans usually falls to younger relatives, close friends, or paid professionals—who also are likely to be confused by the complexity.

Understanding coding and medical billing

After receiving medical services, you can expect to receive bills, statements, and confusing notifications. Many elderly find these notifications incomprehensible, as they are filled with numbers and jargon that list many different kinds of fees already paid, services rendered, and outstanding balances. An accountant can find these codes and bills difficult to understand; for an older person, its complexity is unfair and cruel. It is not clear who is responsible, if there is anyone responsible, to pay the outstanding balance. Have all the medical bills been fully paid, or will subsequent bills be arriving by mail for the remaining balance? If the numbers don't add up, who is being shortchanged?

As you may have noticed, most bills originating from hospitals, medical groups, doctors, et al., come from billing services, sometimes located out of state or even out of country, as is often indicated on their return address. These are computer-generated bills. This adds an extra, impersonal intermediary between you, the patient, and your provider. The bills from the hospitals are the most complicated, because of the complexity of the services that may have been provided. It may seem like "funny money," with charges that appear outrageous, as if in a fantasy board game. There may be charges of tens of thousands of dollars for a one-to-two-day stay; this will stun the average consumer until he or she reads how much balance is remaining after the insurance companies pay their portion. (This also can give you an idea of the cost of medical care today.) If you have an issue with the bill, and believe it's wrong, who do you challenge? That answer is easy—challenge the original provider. They have the clout with their own billing service that you lack. For services where you have no idea of who actually provided the service (e.g., a pathology report), call the primary biller for the service. Bills can be generated for almost any service provided. Mostly they are bundled together. As mentioned above, patients are responsible for dealing with their insurance company. They may not have purchased the insurance coverage that they thought they had, and it is their responsibility to pay the bill if the service was not covered. Usually, the provider checks with the insurance company (sometimes the insurance company even requires preauthorization) to check on the coverage before providing the service.

As mentioned above, the business of medicine is now computer operated. As a result, all services must have specific code numbers for computer input. Every patient has an identification number; every provider (no matter what specialty), every procedure, and every diagnosis have unique identifying numbers. In this way, medical care can be tracked by the patient, the provider, and by what is being done, and for what diagnostic reason. Any inaccurate coding for the diagnosis or the procedure performed will result in an inaccurate fee being paid by the insurance company. If the diagnostic code that accompanied the bill does not seem to justify the procedure (e.g., a laboratory test), the insurance company can refuse to pay for it; this leaves the laboratory or provider left holding the bag. They can then resubmit the bill with another diagnostic code, bill the patient, or absorb the loss.

When Medicare pays a bill or reimburses a patient, the patient receives a statement of the EOB—the explanation of benefits. Despite the efforts of a lot of very intelligent people to make these statements understandable, many patients and families are bewildered and need further explanation. The problem seems to arise from the attempt of the insurance companies to make these statements comprehensive and complete. The result is that there is *too* much information, and this leads to confusion. Included in the statements is the *actual amount* that the provider charged (*not* the DRG [diagnosis related group] amount that insurance companies use to calculate reimbursement), the amount the insurance company allowed, how much they paid as the primary (or secondary) insurance, the amount of deductible outstanding, and how much balance remains. Somewhere on the statement there is a note that the patient is not responsible for paying the remaining balance; this leaves the insured with confusion and the question of who is responsible for the balance that is unaddressed.

It would be a lot simpler if the insurance company just listed what services were billed and how much they paid. Since it is not a bill, the fine details and balance are not really relevant. Perhaps there is a desire to educate the consumer about how much the hospital, laboratory, physician, etc., is really charging (or would have charged), had not the insurance company negotiated a lower fee—they look better to the public if it appears they have helped reduce the public's national health-care costs. The consequence of all these official-looking statements pouring in by mail is that many older people become anxious and uncertain as to how to keep and store these records for possible future need. These statements look very official, and therefore it seems that they should be filed and kept forever, with other important papers.

Nonetheless, a wise consumer should read the statement and make a note of whether the services were really provided and are valid. Frequently they may not recognize the name of the provider, and wonder if the services were billed to them by mistake. Even when the name of the provider is recognized, many patients complain that they receive notice of payment for a service that they can't recall ever being performed. This makes for a difficult scenario. Were these fraudulent charges? Who ordered or performed these services? Were these services really necessary? Accusations of fraud are a serious issue.

Often doctors visit patients in the hospital (perhaps as a consultant) and find the patient in a foggy and not very interactive state, and do not spend much time talking to the patient at the bedside. The patient may not recall ever seeing this provider, or may question whether the service was even necessary. The patient may be right. Alternatively, the provider may be spending considerable time reviewing the hospital chart for laboratory results, notes from other consultants or providers, the medications being given, etc. These activities are being done at the nursing station, or another location away from the patient's direct observation. The services and bill may therefore be valid and justified. The patient should realize that the insurance company is well aware of these issues, and has their own team of experts investigating whether there are any fraudulent charges being made. They see patterns of charges, and are even more concerned than the patient about being overly billed. They can set up audits and investigate legitimacy of the charges the same way the IRS can do to a taxpayer. They can demand a refund from the provider if they believe the charges were unjustified, and have the legal team to back up any legal issues.

Surviving Hospitalization

Hospitals can be dangerous places, particularly for the elderly. Hospitals, also, are not what they used to be. Understanding today's hospitals and hospital routines is the first step toward a satisfactory hospital stay. A fresh understanding may also help you preserve your (and your family's) composure and sanity, and help reduce potential errors in your care. Hospitals have become complex institutions, and complex businesses, with many more types of personnel involved in patient care.

Physicians rarely run hospitals (as they had done decades ago)—business executives now do, and are under the same pressures experienced by any large business or corporation. Salaries for these executives must be competitive with other businesses, and the cost of running the hospital has increased dramatically. These costs eventually get passed on to the patient and the insurance companies. Furthermore, the more complex a medical problem, and the more people involved in patient care, the greater the opportunity for mistakes to occur.

Expect that things may not be done in the hospital the way you think they should. Try to be a partner with your hospital team (not just be a patient or an adversary). Getting better is made easier if everyone involved in your care (you and the staff taking care of you) are on the same page and communicating and working smoothly together. Being helpful and assistive in your own care can be to your benefit.

When hospitalized, here are some rules you should know. The key rules are: to ask questions if there are things you don't understand, or if you think something is being done improperly. But ask your questions and speak to the appropriate person. Obviously, your questions should be framed in a thoughtful rather than an accusatory way. Secondly, have a family advocate. Being a patient, you most likely will be confined to a bed or a hospital chair, with limited awareness of what is happening around you. You also will be preoccupied with being tested, therapies, people asking questions, etc. You need someone who knows you, and can supply hospital staff with information about you that the hospital records may not contain. And you need someone who can observe what is happening with fresh eyes. There is a tendency (see below on maintaining our humanity) to treat patients as chart numbers and "cases." An advocate keeps real your humanity and can keep reminding hospital staff that you are a real person. The advocate also brings a bit of the real, outside world to you, and can keep you informed and oriented to what is happening in the world outside your hospital room. Further, if there is a conflict, your advocate (being healthier and more mobile than you) is in a better position to present your position and fight for your rights.

There are many different professionals and staff in the hospital who will interact with you as a patient. Try to understand what role each is playing in your care. It is very appropriate to ask people who they are and what role they serve, if it is not obvious. In large teaching or academic medical centers, there are people in many different roles who will interact with the patient. Aside from your primary attending doctor, there are nurses: head nurses, floor nurses, and often nursing students. They change with each eight-hour shift, as nurses must be available twenty-four hours/day, seven days a week, and no nurse can work multiple successive shifts. There are nursing aides, who help the nurse, but are not nurses, nor trained as nurses. There are therapists of all sorts: physical therapists, occupational therapists, respiratory therapists, speech, and swallow therapists. There are social workers and discharge planning nurses to help you with your needs and problems in and out of the hospital. There are specialty nurses, such as wound-care nurses. There are nurse-practitioners (more about them in another section). There may be medical students and doctors-in-training (postgraduate training), who are closely involved in determining your care. There may be "teaching" medical attendings (for "teaching" the doctors-in-training —the doctors previously called interns and residents), and "hospitalists" (more about them below). There are specialty teams in surgery, oncology, obstetrics, urology, transplant surgery, pain management, and palliative care. There are housekeeping, dieticians and food delivery, TV maintenance, and equipment maintenance personnel; and there are pharmacists and pharmacy aids, secretaries, clerks and receptionists. As discussed below, most hospitals also employ patient advocates or liaisons to help with specific problems you may have with the care you are receiving in the hospital. There are a lot of people involved in the care of a hospitalized patient—one of the reasons the costs involved in hospital stay are so staggering.

Hospital staff, representing many of these roles, often visits the patient soon after admission, and ask probing questions, and may examine the patient. This can be a source of irritation to the patient, who wonders why people keep asking them the same questions someone else had previously asked. This can be particularly annoying when the newly admitted patient is exhausted, uncomfortable, frightened, sleep-deprived, and not thinking clearly. However, just because on admission they might not be thinking as clearly as when they are more relaxed, on repeated questioning and presenting their story to successive questioners, the history becomes more complete, and important events or connections that were not initially appreciated gain more relevance and importance.

Effective interacting with hospital personnel is a critical aspect of successful hospitalization. Realize that, even with the best of intentions, the hospital personnel sees the older individual as an old patient, while the family sees before them a beloved close member of the family in distress. Despite some differences in perspective, everyone involved should be on the same page and working together with the goal of making the older patient better, and in improving to a status of being able to go home with the admitting problem satisfactorily resolved. Ranting and screaming at the hospital personnel is very counterproductive.

Which hospital, and to what type of hospital a person is admitted, can make a significant difference in the care and outcome of the admitting problem. To begin with, patients may not realize it, but they have a right to choose to which hospital they wish to be admitted and treated. In communities where there are several hospitals or medical centers present, the choice of where an individual wishes to be treated, have surgery, or receive emergency care is an important one, taking many issues into consideration. If taken by EMS to the hospital, the patient may end up in a hospital not of their choosing; but this is only if the EMS team feels that their condition is emergent and requires going to the closest available hospital. Transferring patients from one hospital to another entails problems. Generally, patients cannot be transferred from one hospital's emergency department to another's ED. Once admitted, interhospital transfers require several conditions be met: (1) the patient must request transfer; (2)

the patient must be in stable enough condition to be safely transferred; (3) there must be an accepting physician at the receiving hospital; and (4) there must be a bed available at the accepting hospital that can provide the level of care needed.

Hospitals are not what they were in the past. All patients (as well as their families), but particularly older patients, need to understand some basic aspects of hospital care if they are to survive hospitalization with some degree of composure. First, one must understand that there are different types of hospitals: public, voluntary, and private. Hospitals may be teaching (and training hospitals—connected to teaching medical schools and medical centers), or be purely proprietary. By definition, a voluntary hospital is "a private, not-for-profit hospital that provides uncompensated care to the poor." It is very useful to understand what kind of hospital is being entered, and what type of care the patient will encounter. It should be repeated that most all hospitals now have patient liaisons and patient advocates available to help them with problems that arise during their hospital stay. One needs only to ask for their involvement. Their services are free. There also social workers on staff, who are mandated, at no cost to the patient, to help patients and their families cope with the hospitalization and post-discharge care.

In teaching hospitals (particularly those connected with medical schools), patients may not have their private physician, and will be assigned to a team, where routine medical and surgical care is usually provided by doctors-in-training; that is to say, third- and fourth-year medical students, interns, residents, and fellows (these last are now called PGY-1, -2, -3, etc. [for "postgraduate year" 1, 2, 3, etc.]) PGYs 2 and greater are usually licensed physicians. Attending physicians are assigned to oversee the care, and to teach the junior medical staff. Most often, attending physicians are forbidden by medical center policy to write any orders for care—they must only be written by the PGYs. For many medical problems, having an in-house medical team available twenty-four hours/day, seven days a week, more than compensates for the absence of the private attending physician. Also, one should consider the priorities and agenda that are shared by prestigious teaching medical centers. They may have the perceived best doctors, facilities, and perform the latest advances in medical and surgical care, but this comes at a price. Teaching medical centers must teach students and doctors-in-training; they are heavily involved in medical and basic science research. They grant degrees and certificates of completion of training. Their programs are reviewed regularly to assure that these educational and training programs meet national standards. Although very important, patient care is not the primary objective of these medical centers. Lastly, they must balance their budget; fees for patient care must often subsidize the less-remunerative functions of the medical center. Foreign medical graduates require training as PGYs in US hospitals with approved training programs.

Many public and voluntary hospitals in the US are now hiring "hospitalists" to manage *all* hospitalized patients. Hospitalists are salaried doctors, employed by the hospital. In many parts of the US, this is the rule and not the exception. Other hospitals may have a mixture of patients, some cared for by private attending physicians and others by hospitalists. In these hospitals, only if the patient clearly requests that their private physician (and NOT the hospitalist) manage their case, will this request be granted. If a patient is admitted to a hospitalist, the private attending physician must relinquish all aspects of their care. The hospitalists are assigned on admission. For patients cared for by a hospitalist, the hospitals will bill the insurance companies for both the hospital and professional components of care. Where there are hospitalists, the hospital will likely try to steer all admissions to the care of the hospitalist, as this type of care is more profitable to the hospital. This care may also more efficient, as hospitalists may be more available than the private medical doctor, and can order tests, and start treatment sooner.

In private hospitals, patients have their usually familiar private attending physician who manages all aspects of their hospital stay. These doctors generally know the patient and their families, and what has been done previously. They tend to order fewer tests (as they are familiar with past examinations) and can put complaints into a context of past events.

So why is the hospitalist replacing the private physician in so many hospitals? There are benefits the hospitalist provides to the patient and the hospital. Trained hospitalists are available on site throughout the day to respond to any medical or hospital problem, and can shorten the hospital stay (more about this later). Unlike the private physician with a busy office practice, patients don't have to wait till the private physician can break away to visit the hospitalized patient. Hospitalists may also increase the hospital's revenue. Since medical issues in the hospital do not follow a nine to five schedule five days a week, the presence of hospitalists may allow the hospital to operate without regard to holidays, weekends, or time of day. This puts a greater strain on hospitalists, who probably have families, children, and other personal commitments. It reduces the pool of physicians who would be willing to take on the role of a hospitalist. On the down side, patients lose the comfort of having the physician they know and trust overseeing their care. At a time when they are frightened, or even terrified, about what is happening to them, they are asked to place their full confidence in the hospitalist, who may be a total stranger. This hospitalist will probably not be caring for them after they are discharged, and will have no long-term involvement with them or their family. In situations where there are no hospitalists, residents, or physicians-in-training, a licensed "floating" hospital physician, nurse practitioners (see below), and registered nurses fill in for the absent private physician when needed for emergencies.

Many older patients become confused and disoriented in the hospital —a phenomenon that greatly disturbs their families. The changing environment, the changing faces and names of the staff that care for them, the daily attempts to take blood, the special testing, the disruption of their sleep and daily hospital routines, all tend to put tremendous pressure on their psyche. The patient's psyche is already threatened by the stress of being in the hospital, and the fear of what might be happening in their body and what the future might bring. Awakening patients at four or five a.m. to check their weight is particularly irritating. The need to do this, the hospital argues, is that weights are important, and the staff only have the early morning hours free to check weights before things get too busy later in the morning. Hopefully, newer hospital beds with built-in scales can measure weights at any time, with no disturbance to the patient.

Another disturbing hospital routine is the "portable" X-ray being taken on another patient in a neighboring bed. In this scenario, X-ray technicians come into the room, at any hour, and ask all visitors to leave. All hospital staff also quickly exits the premises, so as not to be exposed to the added radiation. However, the other patients in the environs are not moved. When a patient confined to a nearby bed asks why they are not being shielded, the reply usually is, "It's too little radiation to give you any need for concern." This they hear from the very knowledgeable people who are rushing out of the way so as not to be exposed themselves. The justification for this behavior, it is argued, is that hospital staff would otherwise be exposed repeatedly, on a daily basis, to such radiation. This would have cumulative effects of radiation overexposure over periods of months and years.

Older patients are at risk of immediately losing all sense of individuality and dignity, and become dependent on others for every aspect of their care. Families can help by keeping the patient oriented to place, time, and person. Family visits and support are very helpful. This point cannot be stressed enough. Elderly patients who have no visitors are at a serious disadvantage in the hospital setting. Hospitals can help reduce disorientation by trying to limit moving the patient from room to room and keeping the staff caring for the patient as consistent as possible by trying to limit the numbers of different nurses et al. caring for patients throughout their stay. Patients are moved from one semiprivate room to another when a "male bed" or "female bed" becomes needed by a discharge, since co-ed rooms are not usually allowed except in ICUs and rooms having patients needing specialized care.

Another aspect of hospital care is that, in the hospital, patients are exposed to germs that are usually much more dangerous and much more resistant to antibiotics than they are at home. Resistant germs are encouraged by the wide use of antibiotics in the hospital (antibiotics used to treat resistant germs). Germs come in with the patient in the next bed (you do your share and bring in yours). Visitors, and hospital staff who visit and examine multiple patients, carry germs. For the sake of comfort, reduced stress and pressure on their psyche, and avoidance of hospital-acquired infections, home is much the better environment for an older, frightened person.

How hospitals are paid, and how they encourage shorter lengths of stay (LOS) will be discussed in a later section (Advocacy and Finances).

Differences in Care between Types of Hospitals

PRIVATE OR VOLUNTARY HOSPITAL	TEACHING HOSPITAL
Private physician manages care	Assigned hospitalist manages care

One primary doctor throughout	Risk of multiple "primary" doctors
Pvt. Office hours may delay care	Doctors available 24hrs X 7days,
Consulting specialists chosen	Consulting specialists assigned
Continuity with post discharge	Fragmentation of care
Tendency to treat patient	Tendency to treat disease
Tendency for less testing	Tendency for more testing
Longer stays—less efficient	Shorter stays—more efficient

Struggling with End-of-Life Decisions
Need for care

We hope to have a long lifetime; time enough in which to make plans for when we become ill or too weak to manage our own affairs. Still, with all that time, it's usually a crisis that happens, and plans must suddenly be made. This can occur after an accident, a stroke, or a loss of a supportive care-partner. As with disability or life insurance, we may wish never to need them, but it is prudent to have contingency plans.

With serious illness, patients or their families should anticipate that a medical team will present them with a series of choices regarding end-of-life care. They will ask the patient (or their health proxy) to sign documents regarding limiting end-of-life care (see DNR and DNI below). These are very emotional decisions, and will cause stress and hesitation—and, if unprepared, much anxiety and second-guessing. Too often the person agreeing with the proposed plan of care begins to question their decision after several hours, discusses his or her decision with other family members, and spreads the anxiety throughout their circle of close contacts. I recommend that unless prepared and firm in one's attitude toward end-of-life care, the individual should defer and sleep on his or her decision overnight before signing any agreement. It's also helpful to have other family members present, when these choices are presented and explained, to prevent any later misunderstandings. Remember, too, that patients are allowed to change their mind and reverse previously made decisions.

Assuming we don't die, but need more help with our basic needs, we should be prepared and have considered all the options. If we need additional help, should we have this while still living in our homes? Should we move to an "assisted living" arrangement, where we have an individual apartment but live in a place where there are trained people around who can help us if we need assistance? Would we need to be in an institution, such as a nursing home, where there is more intensive nursing available? Should we consider places where there are multiple levels of care, where we can move from one level to another, as our needs change? Should we stay near our children and family, or move to a climate that is less harsh and severe than where we currently reside? And how will we pay for this? Do we need "long-term health-care insurance" (as described above, p. 196)? These are all valid questions that need serious consideration and family discussion. A wise attitude is to be prepared for all contingencies.

There may come a time, when the disease burden or the breakdown of so many organs and functions in the debilitated individual is too great to sustain life, when the patient enters into a phase of dying. Doctors may recognize this (and the patients may too), but families frequently do not. This happens most often in patients being cared for in hospital intensive care units or ICUs. Families may ask for "everything to be done." Doctors may alternatively be suggesting "palliative care." The latter type of care is aimed at providing "comfort measures" only, and not treating the underlying disease, which doctors feel is no longer treatable. The goal is to allow the person to die in peace and with dignity.

Families often become very concerned about feeding measures and fluids. As discussed above, there are the issues of feeding tubes, placed through the nose or directly into the stomach through the abdominal wall. There also are choices of intravenous feeding and fluids. For patients who are dying, or making their advance directives, these issues of feeding and IVs also need to be addressed. Patients and health proxies can also request no blood drawing or IVs be given, to halt all testing, and to limit care to only that which will relieve pain and stress. The guiding principal should be whether any of these measures would benefit the patient. Can the individual experience any further pleasure or quality of life? Is death just being postponed, or can more aggressive therapy be justified?

News media sometimes publicize an extraordinary case of an individual for whom all hope for survival had vanished, but who miraculously survived. This story gives renewed hope for miracles to happen for all families of patients who are dying, the hope that if the patients could only be kept alive indefinitely, maybe they would recover. There is, however, a difference between living and merely existing; the former implies some aspect or hope for an iota of human cognitive activity. If there is no hope for recovery of meaningful life, what is being accomplished by keeping a body alive by extraordinary measures? These issues are no longer medical, but rather religious and philosophical, and doctors have no greater wisdom or authority than anyone else. Availability of ICU beds is finite and limited, and keeping patients in ICUs while awaiting miracles prevents the beds and space being used for patients who can be treated and helped by the intensive medical and nursing care of the ICU. Other patients are thus deprived of the ICU care because of lack of beds. There consequently can be friction between the families and the health providers in the hospital. Most hospitals have ethicists and clergy, along with social workers and administrators, to help discuss the situation with the family and medical staff, and focus discussion onto realistic expectations.

Hospice care is offered to individuals with limited life expectancy (usually anticipated to be six months or less). Hospice care can be provided either at the person's home (outpatient) or at a hospice institution (inpatient). As with palliative care, hospice care is aimed at comfort care only, not managing the primary disease. The patient usually suffers from terminal malignancy, but many hospices do not require a cancer diagnosis. Hospices generally have staff personnel available to assist the patient with help at all times, including nights, holidays, and weekends; they are excellent with pain control and emotional support. There are also a variety of community services and institutions available to provide support and help for patients and families with cancer diagnoses (e.g., Cancer Care; Gilda's Club). The American Cancer Society is a good contact resource for what services are available.

It often is very helpful to consult an elder lawyer. Elder lawyers can advice families how best to protect their assets, and explain their rights. One should consider the services of an elder lawyer before any crises develop, if problems can be anticipated. Early planning is much better than end panic.

Health-care agencies can be employed to assist patients who wish to remain at home. They have the means to provide any and all support the patient might need (nurses, home attendants, therapists, testing, durable appliances, etc.). Agencies vary in their charges to the patient, and in what ancillary services they can provide. A prudent approach is to be a cautious shopper, and evaluate several agencies before making a choice.

Understanding and making advance directives

No matter how much we may dislike thinking about our end-of-life or terminal care, it's an issue that eventually will need to be addressed. There is a need to have "advance directives." These documents are generally referred to as a living will and a health proxy. One does not need a lawyer to draw up these documents.

When people die, and the heart stops beating and the lungs stop breathing, there generally was an underlying reason. Success at resuscitation will depend upon that reason. Reestablishing a heartbeat or breathing does not change the underlying conditions in the individual. In some cases, the immediate cause for death (such as an infection, bleeding, or trauma) is amenable to treatment; in other cases, if given more time, the body can "compensate" and adjust to a new problem such as a stroke, heart attack, or embolus. However, in most cases the death of the individual is a result of the body no longer being able to sustain itself, and resuscitation will be futile.

An individual always has the right to choose what therapy he or she wishes, or does not wish, to accept. The difficulties arise when a person is not able to direct his or her care, due to being unconscious or incapacitated in a way that makes him or her less able to give reliable informed consent for treatment. A living will merely gives an indication of an individual's general philosophy regarding end-of-life decisions (e.g., willingness to accept respirators—being intubated with a tube into the lung and attached to a ventilator, resuscitation, feeding tubes, etc.). There are such things as "time-dependent" living wills, in which a person may agree to such measures and devices, but only for a limited period of time. If there is improvement in the condition, these measures can be continued, but if the outlook looks hopeless, they direct such "artificial" measures be discontinued.

Patients are now being asked more frequently their views regarding DNR and DNI (Do Not Resuscitate, and Do Not Intubate). Discussion of end-of-life decisions usually makes people uncomfortable, and they may not fully understand what is being offered. A DNR order is not an order to withhold or not provide any treatment. A DNR merely means that should the person die (i.e., they stop breathing and their heart stops beating), attempts will not be made to resuscitate them. Some patients and families opt for "limited" resuscitation: a single attempt to restore breathing and heartbeat. A DNI order means that if the individual has trouble breathing, they do not wish to have a tube inserted into their trachea and be attached to a ventilating machine. This is usually an issue only if it is felt that the ventilator (an artificial breathing machine) will be needed for the remaining lifetime of the patient.

A health proxy names an individual who speaks for the patient—speaking with the patient's voice, not their own. This requires that the named health proxy (who has permission only to make health-matter decisions for the patient) be fully aware of the attitudes toward health care held by the patient. A health proxy can override any wishes expressed in a living will, and is the more important of the two documents. The patient's physician cannot also be the health proxy. Otherwise, the health proxy can be anyone whom the patient trusts, relative or nonrelative.

It should be clear from the discussion of this section and the previous section that all people should understand what is happening to their bodies and what health care is about. They should have realistic expectations, and discuss their feelings with their family and those close to them, particularly those who might have to help them make life-involving decisions. It is important that these documents be available in an emergency, and that the means to contact the health proxy be clearly outlined.

Considering of end-of-life choices is a bit like considering life insurance—it's emotionally uncomfortable, and we would rather be thinking about other things. Know that all advance directives can be changed or rescinded. Having ambivalence is very common, and older patients frequently change their minds about what care they would, or would not, prefer. But it is their choice, and they should not be cajoled into choosing what the doctor or staff recommends. They and their family need to understand, in the most objective way, what choices are available. They may want to ask more questions, or discuss the issues with their clergy, or with people they trust.

Teaming and Interacting with Your Doctor
Hiring a doctor

Everyone wants "the best doctor"! And who is the "best doctor": the one with the most elegant office—the one charging the highest fees in the best neighborhood—the one written up in a magazine—the one with the most celebrities as patients—the one who graduated or trained at a prestigious institution? I would maintain that there is no "best doctor." *Best doctor* is a relative term—the best doctor for whom? Someone else's best doctor may not be the best doctor for you. The best primary-care doctor for any individual patient is one who has a good base of current medical knowledge, has an inquisitive mind and keeps learning, listens to the patient and communicates effectively with him, respects the patient and has his best interests always foremost in their recommendations; the best doctor has a network of colleagues who are respected in their field, and whose work habits and location meet the patient's needs. Best doctors are those who are not embarrassed to say, "I don't know" and are willing to call for help.

In choosing surgeons or specialists, it is best to ask for recommendations from your primary-care doctor or to pick a physician working at an institution where you might want to have the specialty care or surgery. Many of my patients choose specialists by researching the individual physician on the Internet. Remember, you are not only choosing a physician, you are choosing a complete package of care for that malady. For major surgery, you are choosing an institution: an anesthesiologist, a recovery room staff, postoperative nursing, rehabilitation etc.—a lot more than just a surgeon. Further, if you want good communication between your primary care doctor and the specialty care, it is best that they can easily and comfortably communicate between each other. This is best done when they know each other and can easily contact each other by phone, face to face, or by e-mail, Twitter, texting, etc.

Unfortunately, the best-made plans often go astray. We live in a world of managed care. Patients carefully investigate which physicians are on their plan, only to discover that the physician has since dropped out of that insurance network. Often, patients select a plan specifically for the purpose of retaining a particular physician as their primary-care doctor. But there is no obligation that the physician continues to participate with the plan, and if reimbursement rates or logistics make participation less desirable for the physician, he or she will drop out. Sometimes, it is hard to get referrals to specialists who are participating in the network, despite what the primary-care doctor accepts. This often leads to frustration and problems in the delivery of care. Things might work out better if the primary doctor functions in a multispecialty group, where everyone associated with the group participate in the same plans. As discussed below, some patients choose two sets of doctors to manage their care.

Then there is the hospital. Does it participate in your insurance plan, and which hospital does the individual wish to have as their hospital? In some communities there is no choice; in others there are many choices. But when choosing a doctor, aside from the individual characteristics of that physician, it is wise to consider also with which hospital they are affiliated, and who covers for the doctor when he or she is away; who does the doctor usually select for specialty consultations? Nothing is written in stone, and situations change, but at the very least, these issues should be considered before choosing a doctor. Some individuals will make an appointment to screen the doctor—to see if they mesh, and have a good rapport and share a similar attitude regarding health and dying. It is also important to have a sense of where the doctor's primary allegiance lies: with the patient or with the insurance company, hospital, or group that pays his or her salary.

In today's world, doctors are often limited in how much time they can spend with a patient. This is particularly true in clinics and managed-care practices. Older people generally need more time with the doctor than do younger people. They may need repetitive explanations till they understand what is being said. The elderly person generally processes information slower, moves slower, and has a lot more problems and worrisome issues. Because older patients generally take more physician time during an office visit, and because the elderly may not have an insurance that reimburses or pays the doctor as well as some other insurance company, many doctors try not to accept too many elderly patients into their practice. Being aware of this fact can reduce a lot of anger and resentment (see section below on "Cooperative Interacting with Your Doctor").

But it should be remembered that your doctor is there for you, the patient; the patient is not there for the doctor. You essentially are hiring the doctor, and you are really "the boss" (but don't push this point too hard).

Cooperative interacting with your doctor

Older patients can help themselves by reflecting on what really is bothering them and by going to the doctor's office prepared:

ready to discuss what it is that really bothers them most. Going through a long laundry list of every complaint they had experienced the preceding several months with the doctor is counterproductive. You do not bring your old car to the mechanic complaining of every dent, stain, and scratch (otherwise prepare for leaving your car there for months, and expect an enormous bill). As with the old car, there will always be something wrong; the focus should be on the top two or three complaints that are appropriate. Going through the "laundry list" also marks the patient as being incapable of differentiating what is important and what is not. Although you may feel unable to judge the significance of each and every complaint, prioritize, and stick to the top two to three issues that concern you, starting with what bothers you most. You may find the doctor stops your listing of complaints after the first two or three items, and before you had even gotten to your major concern, if you had planned to bring it up late in the visit. Alternatively, you may notice the doctor's eyes glaze over when you get to your fifth complaint. And don't assume that your doctor remembers all your test results and everything in your medical history without consulting your medical record, or that your doctor has been discussing your case with all the other professionals involved in your care. You have only one person to consider, but the doctor probably has many patients with similar complaints and may need reminding of your particular situation.

Doctors cannot simply connect your body to a computer to see what's wrong with you. Unless the cause is obvious, working up a complaint may be very involved, costly, and uncomfortable. In presenting your problem (your history), try to be as clear and precise as possible. Some words—*dizzy, tired, sick,* and *weak*—are too vague to be used in a medical setting without more clarification.

There is a limit to how many tests and treatments can be initiated at one time. The more complaints you present, the more testing and more consulting doctor visits you may be asked to undertake. This is another reason to prioritize your concerns. Excessive testing overwhelms the individual. Focusing only on top priorities means these top complaints will be addressed. Eventually, persisting or bothersome complaints (those lower on the priority list of problems) will have their turn.

The person should consider the net benefit to their life if any particular condition were reversed. How would their life be better? Would it be worth risking the penalties of an intensive workup and treatment? A minimal benefit may not make medical attention worthwhile, and a high-risk procedure, which would extend their life by only several weeks, may not be worth doing. Only the individual knows how much each complaint really bothers them.

Having a medley of specialists caring for each of the patient's organ systems often compounds this difficulty. Each specialist rightly focuses on his or her area of greatest interest, and orders tests and procedures as if this problem alone is the one that needs attention. To the specialist, any issue involving their area of expertise is a priority. Someone needs to be looking after the patient as a whole. After all, most would agree that caring doctors should be treating the patient, not the disease or the complaint.

When the older patient was younger, there probably was a family doctor, who, in his private office, did everything from delivery of babies, to pediatrics, to minor surgery, to caring for the older sick patient, and who made house calls. Those days are mostly gone, and the expectations that accompanied that kind of health delivery are also obsolete. There are some doctors who still make house calls, but in today's modern medical system, they can provide only limited help for simple, straightforward conditions. For more complicated problems, which are far more common in the elderly, doctors frequently require the assistance of laboratories, radiology, and surgical or neurological consultations. Having a home visit by a physician bringing nothing more than a stethoscope and blood pressure machine can delay diagnostic and treatment opportunities by many, many hours. It may be convenient, but it carries some risk if the individual is really sick.

Also, in the "old days," there was close rapport between doctor and patient. The doctor was like a member of the family, and knew all the family members by name. There was trust and a good relationship. In today's medicine, general family doctors are rare in cosmopolitan regions, and are becoming rare everywhere. We live in a world of specialization, with insurance and hospital-based medical care. The patient and their family must remember that for most doctors, they are not extensions of the health-insurance company. If patients and families are upset about the high cost of their insurance, or problems getting reimbursement, they should NEVER take it out on the physician. To most doctors, the insurance is the patient's business; doctors are there to treat the medical problems and don't want to get involved in insurance issues. They are not employees of the insurance company. Filling out forms, writing letters, and filling out more forms authorizing services, supplies, and government payments are time-consuming (particularly if it requires reviewing the patient's chart) and are not reimbursed. These are things the doctor is doing for the patient's benefit, behind their back. To have that same patient getting angry or upset with the doctor makes the doctor wish that patient would find another doctor. Venting to the doctor about the long wait in the doctor's office, a person who arrived after you going in ahead of you, complaining about the office staff, or asking the doctor to fill out forms, takes away time from your visit, and slows the doctor up even more for the next patient. It becomes a snowball effect. Your doctor may become so distracted in defending or explaining the reason for the delay that your office visit is wasted on this issue alone.

Drop them a note, or send them an e-mail to get your feelings off your chest, while not slowing down the doctor and the office patient flow even further. You always have a choice in changing your doctor.

Being a good patient means helping your doctor take care of you (see the section above on Making Priorities and Life Choices for Healthy Living). Having a primary-care doctor who you trust to help guide you through the labyrinth of complex medical care is very helpful and reassuring. Doctors take their cues from their patients. The more the patient complains about different maladies, the more inclined the doctor will be to prescribe remedies for each. This can result in a large number of referrals and specialists to be seen, many more tests, as well as the accumulation of massive numbers of pills to take each day. Again, my recommendation is to be prepared for the visit, and limit the numbers of complaints to the most important two or three that disturb you the most. If there is an issue that bothers you and you know it will take more time, make that the sole issue for the visit, and offer to come again another time to deal with the other important problems.

Being a good patient and medical consumer also requires being considerate, kind to, and dealing appropriately with the doctor and the hospital or office staff. Most patients realize that the doctor's time is valuable, and that doctors have their own lives and families. Telephone calls are a major point of irritation for both the patient and the doctor. A busy doctor may have as many as twenty to thirty telephone calls a day from patients who request a call back. Before calling to speak to the doctor, you should ask yourself whether the call is *really* necessary; whether you can figure out the answer to your question yourself—or is it that you just want to talk to your doctor? When patients requesting a call back for "test results" are really asking for a telephone consultation, a general discussion of their health, or a mini-course in physiology and medicine, doctors will generally ask their nurse or secretary to call them back or fax them the results, thus avoiding the long conversations.

Sometimes patients call their primary physician to have the doctor explain what another physician had said, or results of tests ordered by another physician; this commonly occurs when the patient does not want to annoy that other doctor, or can't understand their explanations. To develop a good relationship with your doctor, some points should be followed: (1) be prepared with what questions you wish to ask during a requested telephone call-back, and have the list available, not in another room to which you have to go and begin a search. (2) Keep the questions and discussion brief and relevant. If a long explanation is wanted, offer to come to the office and make an appointment. Most doctors do not charge for their telephone time, and long phone calls are unfair. (3) Recognize that if a holiday is coming up, if the doctor is about to leave on a vacation, or is just returning from a vacation, a lot of people may be calling the office about problems more serious than yours. Perhaps it would be best if you called several days earlier or later, when the doctor will be less rushed and frenetic. (4) Bring another person along with you for the doctor's visit (a third person may hear something said that you did not, and can explain what they thought the doctor meant). A nervous and anxious person may not be hearing all that is being said at the time of the visit. Sometimes the other person can even bring up issues that you had forgotten, and can make the visit more productive. (5) Select a family member to be the health contact for your doctor, if you wish your doctor to talk to a family member. And you must give permission to the doctor or staff to discuss this with a family member. Your medical information is private, and it is a violation of your privacy (and of the law) to discuss your medical condition with anyone who does not have your permission to share it. If you have a large family, it is unfair to ask your doctor to discuss your case with every family member who calls his or her office with concerns about your health.

If your doctor generally runs late, and you have to spend a good deal of unexpected waiting time to be seen, you have several choices: bring some reading material, or work to keep yourself occupied until you are called; ask about having the first or last appointment of the day; do not make other timed appointments on the day of your scheduled doctor's appointment (as with a car service or second appointment), so that you won't be getting upset and worried if you are running late. The agitation of waiting raises your blood pressure and gets your mind off the main medical issues that you needed to address. Doctors who work strictly by the clock are generally much more efficient and follow the appointment schedule. The trade-off, of course, is that when your visit comes, don't expect to have a relaxed visit where you can discuss all of your concerns or get explanations of why things are happening. You may find your visit terminated when the time runs out. Decide which kind of a doctor you want.

Being an informed patient and smarter consumer

Being a good patient also means being a good historian. Most of the information a doctor uses to make a diagnosis comes from the patient's history. This is a crucial element in determining what is going on. To be a good historian, patients need to anticipate the questions that any medical or health personnel may ask about their complaints: "Have you ever had these symptoms before?" "What was happening when the event occurred?" "How did it start, were there any advance warning signs or premonitory feelings; how severe was it; how long did it last?" "Did you find anything that gave you relief, or that made it worse?" "Was there any fever, sweating, nausea associated with the symptoms?" If there is any pain, the patient can look for signs of inflammation—any tenderness, warmth, swelling, or redness? These are all clues to what is going on, and the answers will be very helpful in making a diagnosis.

Patients frequently present their complaints in a biased manner, colored by their own interpretations and diagnoses. For example, a woman might say, "I'm having gallbladder pain." The proper presentation should be free of diagnostic interpretation, such as, "I'm having abdominal pain." By giving their personal diagnosis to the symptoms, the patient may influence the doctor's thinking and limit the possible workup. Let the doctor make the interpretation and diagnosis—that's why you went to see the doctor in the first place. The "gallbladder pain" may be coming from any number of causes. Ascribing it to the gallbladder may create a mind-set that is too restricted. Patients should report their symptoms clearly, completely, and as objectively as possible, without editorial comment. It is OK to present the complaint with an addendum such as, "Could this be coming from the gallbladder?" But the patient should not try to limit the possible diagnostic thinking. The patient is no doubt trying to be helpful, show their medical sophistication, and speed the workup along by their interpretation, but it can be counterproductive. When doctors become patients, they are very careful not to diagnose themselves.

It is very useful to learn how to feel one's own pulse. This can be done easily, with a little practice, by gently feeling over the inside of the wrists, the front/side of the neck, the temple, or below the inner anklebone. One can then measure the heart rate by counting the beats in thirty seconds and multiplying by two. The strength of the pulse can also give a clue as to how good the circulation is to these areas. Pay particular attention to the regularity, the rate, and the strength of the pulse. If a person is dizzy, or is having trouble breathing, it is important to note what the heart is doing, and how the person is breathing at that time: is the heart rate very irregular, can the pulse be felt, is the person sweaty, pale, or nauseated; how is the breathing? This information should be written down and relayed to the appropriate health-care person first seeing the patient.

It is also very important for the older person, and their family, to have realistic expectations of the disease being treated. An open and frank discussion of the different party's expectations for recovery and function will get people on the same page, and avoid much grief, anger, and disappointment. Being too pessimistic about a medical condition, or being too Pollyanna and optimistic, is not advisable. Neither extreme deals with the reality of the situation, and is doomed to cause problems.

Older persons should also be proactive, and tell the physician their views regarding life and death. If doctors uses jargon or initials that patients do not understand, they should ask for a translation. Patients should never be afraid to reveal their ignorance about health matters. It is their body, and they have every right to know what's going on in it, explained in terms they can understand. For the physician, it is always good to know the views of the patient. The best health care always involves both the physician and the patient—it is a team effort. Just as important as it is to have a good doctor, it is important to be a good patient. The latter requires that patients understand what is being asked of them, understand medical instructions, and ask questions if they don't understand.

Managing medical emergencies

Sooner or later medical emergencies occur. Since there are 168 hours in a week, and most medical offices are open only forty hours per week, the likelihood that a random emergency will occur when the medical office is open will be less than one-fourth of the time (even less when we count in the holidays). Most emergencies will therefore occur when the office is closed.

Then there is the issue of where the doctor and your preferred hospital are located. Often the doctor you have chosen, or the hospital or medical center you wish to provide your emergency room or inpatient care, are located some distance from where you live, work, or spend your time. This leads to confusion and anxiety at a time when the individual is already stressed with an acute emergency. Calling 911 or the EMS brings emergency assistance, but they may not take you to where you had wanted to go. The EMS staff is trained to evaluate the condition of the patient, and, if they think it's perilous, they are instructed to take the individual to the closest hospital emergency department that is receiving patients. Transferring from one hospital to another was discussed above (see Surviving Hospitalization).

It pays to have advance planning. Some patients have two or more sets of doctors that they regularly see: one, a local community physician to manage the more common and general medical conditions; and a second doctor they see once or twice a year in order to have that doctor involved in their case when difficult issues arise. That second doctor is usually selected by the affiliation to the hospital or medical center in which the patient wishes to receive any sophisticated or complicated health care. If the older person spends winter in one location and summer in another, they may have "teams" of doctors scattered all over the country. If there are several sets of doctors managing a patient's care, it is vital that each understands and agrees with the care the other is providing, and patients should assure that laboratory test results, lists of current medications, etc., are sent to each doctor. This essentially places the task of managing the medical managers on the patient and the family. It is a good idea to ask for copies of test results, and lists of current medications taken; these can then be shown to whichever doctor the patient sees. Do not expect the multiple doctors to coordinate their schedules to discuss your case. As discussed below, we are entering an era of paperless charts, where all medical information will be stored in electronic health records (EHR). Eventually these records will be accessible from any medical office having your permission. This will allow better coordination of care regardless of where you travel, and which doctors you visit.

The old Boy Scout motto of "be prepared" certainly applies to emergency situations. As with other types of emergencies that can happen in your life (e.g., fires or power outages), a plan of what to do in case of a medical emergency is important. Advanced planning is important, and you should have lists of whom to call and what to do written in a place you can easily find. As discussed in a previous section, you may not be as levelheaded and capable of making the right decisions at the moment of the emergency.

Current and Future Issues in Health Care
Advocacy and allegiance

The relationship between a doctor and a patient has remained the same since the earliest times. Alone together, it is still an issue of one person needing medical help, and the other doing the best he or she can, with the knowledge, experience, and tools at hand. What has changed now is the addition of layers of bureaucracy, paperwork, protocols, and regulations imposed by our system. It is important that the patient understand what pressures are exerted on their "health team" (the doctor, insurance company, hospital, pharmacy, etc.). As explained above, physicians may not always be chosen by the patient, but rather "assigned" by the hospital or medical clinic administration. No matter how conscientious and well-meaning a person or institution may be, they still need to pay salaries and make enough profit to stay in business. The adage "The people who pay the bills are the ones who call the shots" is not too far off the mark. The insurance companies pay the bills, and they now dictate how medical care is to be provided. The individual who understands the pressures and reality of the health-care system will be a better consumer.

Patients rightly expect and demand that their welfare be the top priority and concern of everyone involved in their care. They sometimes feel they are being pushed out of the hospital prematurely. What most individuals do not appreciate is that insurance companies no longer reimburse hospitals on the basis of the actual bills and costs being generated. Rather, to encourage lower costs for the insurance carrier, hospitals are reimbursed by the diagnosis, the diagnosis-related group (DRG), with modifiers based on the age of the patient, number of serious comorbid conditions, etc. This essentially means that the hospital will receive a fixed amount of money from the insurance company for an admitted patient, based on the given diagnosis (made at the time of discharge) whether the patient is hospitalized for two days or for twenty. Long hospitalizations therefore lose money for the hospital. Hospitals are under increasing pressure to reduce patient length of stay (LOS).

Hospitals are now losing money, and many hospitals have been forced to close due to financial burdens. Many individuals are still uninsured, or underinsured, and hospitals cannot easily turn critically ill patients away based upon their lack of insurance. Furthermore, in order to be paid by the insurance carrier, the hospital must meet the requirements of the insurance company and show the patient required hospitalization for every billed day they received acute active medical care. The hospital reimbursement system also penalizes hospitals if patients are readmitted too quickly for the same diagnosis (within thirty days of discharge). This discourages hospitals from sending patients home before they are able to be cared for outside of the hospital. Early discharge, however, does shift some of the burden of care to the patient's family. Acute care hospitals are not convalescent institutions or nursing homes. Their primary motivation must be to stay in business, which they will not be able to do if they continually lose money.

The public should realize that economics now drives the medical engine. If, in the hospital or in a medical office, some performed activity doesn't make sense, it probably means it makes a profit. If something that makes sense and seems logical is not done, it probably means it will lose revenue.

This then often leads to problems with older patients in the hospital. Older patients generally have longer stays, due to multiple medical and social problems that engulf them. As they stay in the hospital, they may develop a feeling of comfort and security with their team of doctors and nurses, and are frightened with the idea of leaving this secure environment. Families may be afraid of what might happen at home, during the night or weekend when there is no doctor readily available. But the hospital environment is not always the safest environment. Because of the many patients receiving antibiotics in the hospital, the germs that are found in the hospital are usually "super germs," resistant and unable to be killed by many of the more common antibiotics. Staying in the hospital runs the risk of getting infected with one of these types of bacteria. In addition, staying in the hospital is not really living. Really living is being in your home, surrounded with the people and things you enjoy, and doing the things you want, when you want. The hospital is an artificial world, and is not the ideal spot to spend one's life, particularly when you are old, and time becomes more precious.

Finances control the health-care system

Costs of health care have skyrocketed, and a good portion of national budgets, as well as consumer budgets goes into health care—everywhere in the world. Health care and health insurance is very expensive. So why is US health care so expensive? Over the past decades, management and delivery of health care has changed from a simple and very personal relationship between a patient and his doctor, with the occasional involvement of a local physician-run hospital, to a massive multicomponent industry. Now many very large corporations and syndicates are involved in managing every aspect of health care, even ownership and management of some hospitals. Each large company has its divisions and subdivisions, which are staffed by executives with highly competitive salaries. Each manages massive budgets and oversees many personnel. The corporations, with their stockholders and executives want higher profits from a system that previously had been considered a service profession, where profits were secondary to the prime purpose of helping the patient. Health care is now recognized (if properly managed) as a potentially profitable big business.

Delivery of medical care is also very labor intensive, with many people involved in a single person's care. Each of these people require a salary and benefits. Technology has brought great medical advances, but with a price tag. Everyone wants the best, the most effective, and the latest advanced care. This care is expensive. There is a lot of discussion of how the US health-care system compares to other systems around the world. Are we overpaying for the care we get? One must recognize that there is no country or health care system that can provide *everything* for *everybody*. As soon as one recognizes this reality, the next question will be, "How is health care then to be rationed?" To ration health care, does one use age cutoffs, choose which diseases to treat, which treatments are too expensive; ration by availability of procedures, or by location and neighborhood? Should we ration by how much the person is willing to pay, or limit how much money is available for health care? There is no perfect system. As a side note, when comparing the costs of health care in the US with other countries, it is important to realize that the cost of medical education is subsidized heavily in other countries and graduates of medical schools in these other countries do not graduate with tens of thousands of dollars in debt that needs to be repaid. Secondly, most other developed countries have some kind of "socialized medicine," where, unlike the US, taxpayer money pays for much of medical care.

Another problem with our health-care system is the over-use of the emergency room. Hospital emergency rooms must be staffed twenty-four hours/day, every day: holiday and weekends notwithstanding. The staffing not only includes doctors and nurses, but also radiology, laboratory services, administrative staffs, cleaning and utility staff, et al. Whether one person comes in, or a bus full of injuries comes in, they must be prepared for anything. The cost of operating the ER is enormous, and is largely the same regardless of how many emergencies they see. The cost to the insurance companies is therefore high. Emergency department care is considered the most expensive form of medical care out there. Individuals who have no health insurance or personal doctor, frequently use the emergency room as their primary care health facility—and the rest of us pay for this, one way or another.

When doctors tell patients, "Go to the emergency room," it is much more costly than if the patient were seen in the office. Many facilities are now setting up "Urgent Care" rooms for individuals who can "walk in" without any appointment for an acute problem (but not an emergency one). An illness that has been dragging on for days can be seen in Urgent Care, during defined hours, rather than in an ER. The Urgent Care facility need not be prepared for treating anything that can happen—anytime—the way the ER must. The Urgent Care center may have more limited hours of operation.

Another reason for the high cost of medical care in this country is the practice of "defensive medicine." Because of the concern about being sued for not doing every test, tests are sometimes done for legal purposes, or just in case an issue later arises. The test or procedure is really not needed, but for potential legal issues the tests are ordered. Someone is paying for these tests and procedures.

The challenge of defending our humanity

As Dorothy said in *The Wizard of Oz*, "We're not in Kansas anymore!" We're not in the world of medicine as it was practiced fifty years ago. Computers have changed everything. Computers and science have brought amazing advances in medical care, but at a price. As I have taught medical students over the years, "Computers treat diseases, not patients; doctors should treat patients, not diseases"! "The secret in caring for patients is to start off by caring for patients"! Computers don't care for patients.

Decades ago, before the days of Medicare, there existed limited health insurance coverage (mostly provided by purchase from Blue Cross/Blue Shield). Medical care was a very personal relationship between the patient and the doctor. Who would have thought that such a unique, historic, and trusting relationship could ever become impersonal. However, once Medicare, large private insurance companies, and big business became involved in health care, medical care was doomed to become less personal, and managed in a more corporate manner.

It was inevitable that computers would have an impact on health care, as they already have on virtually every other aspect of our lives. Initially, insurance, hospital management, and supplies were obvious areas where computers would make a lasting and efficient impact in medical care. However, the actual delivery of health care at the very personal, "bedside" treatment level was thought to be outside the venue of computers. After all, how could computers (at least in their current state of technology) deal with the incredibly complex situations encountered when trying to help patients and families deal with an illness? This is what we are now finding out—and there are problems.

"I need a doctor!" This is one of the most common reasons new patients come to see me in my office. What is it they complain about with their previous doctors?

- "My doctor spent more time interacting with his computer than with me."
- "I don't think I ever saw his face; I only saw the back of his head."
- "My doctor never talked to me."
- "My doctor never answered my phone calls."
- "My doctor always seemed to be rushing me out."
- "My doctor didn't seem interested in me."
- "My doctor just kept sending me to see more doctors and sending me for more tests."
- "My doctor was never available—he always seemed to be on vacation or out of town."

If one examines this list of complaints about their prior doctor, one is struck by the realization that these were the very qualities and services that had been provided by the "old fashioned" doctor who cared for the older patient at an earlier time. These are the values they miss in the current medical system, and what they still hope to find in their primary-care doctor.

Computers have already made a big impact on the practice of medicine, and will make a bigger impact in the coming years. Electronic health records (EHR) are being required in all aspects of health care, wherever there is a health provider. At present, there are many different computer and Internet-based programs, but the government is demanding they all be compatible with one another. The goal is to have all medical records (hospital and office) be electronic (paper charts are being retired and becoming a thing of the past). The benefits of EHR are that any patient's medical record can be accessed from anywhere in the country, or maybe the world (this includes what medicines they are taking, the patient's medical history, their physical exams, their X-rays, EKGs, and laboratory results). This will reduce redundancy in testing, and avoid errors in prescribing medicines to which a person is allergic, or which are incompatible with medicines already being taken. All prescriptions will be sent electronically to the pharmacy, reducing errors caused by pharmacists being unable to read the doctor's handwriting. Patients will be able to access their record to view their laboratory results, make or change appointments, or communicate electronically with the office or clinic. The benefits to insurance companies and government is that they can get a better understanding of what is happening between the patient and caregiver at the level of service. They acquire information they want regarding the justification for any ordered tests or procedures. The downside of EHR is the interposition of a computer program between the doctor and the patient. It further separates the doctor from the patient, and tends to make a complex patient fit into a fixed computer program.

Already, every time a test is done, a treatment performed, and a prescription written, a computer identifies the patient, who ordered the test, what test or procedure was done, and what the diagnosis is. Everything has a number. A growing trend in medical centers is to "bar code" the patient on their wristband. This can reduce errors of giving the wrong medicine to the patient, and can improve "tracking," even if it may make the patient feel a bit like a box of cereal. All this information can be collated in computers to follow every aspect of a patient's care. This can be helpful, but also harmful. There's no humanity in the equation. People are different from one another. Diagnoses are only names. Each diagnosis comes in a broad spectrum of severity, and in a wide variation of how it affects the patient and the family. Different patients may have different manifestations of the same diagnosis; diseases can present in a different manor and can affect patients differently. Family situations, home situations, religious convictions, monetary situations, educational difference all impact on medical and social needs. Past experiences and fears all make us who we are, and effect how we react. The computer (at this stage in its use) cannot accept all the subtleties and complexities that go into a person's needs, and which should be considered in their medical care. The value of computerized patient records is very evident—but it must be balanced with the value of the human factors.

To maintain our humanity, it is important for the patient (and the patient's family) to resist being a number, insist on being called by their name, and to advocate for their human needs. If you feel you are being treated as a number, there's nothing wrong with speaking out and reminding your health providers that you are a real person, with complex personal, family, and medical issues. You must be proactive politically and medically, defending your human rights as an individual and as a patient. You can expect resistance from the "system," as adding a human dimension is not programmed into the system the way it once was, and the way we might want. Without causing too much havoc in the medical community, humans should still advocate for our humanity; maybe future health care will reach a new equilibrium in which there will be more of a human element. Alternatively, you can return to the older, more personal private relationship that existed before the days of health insurance, and see a private doctor who does not participate in any insurance plan (see below, p. 238).

Making an extended appointment with your doctor for the primary purpose of keeping in touch can be very helpful in maintaining a personal relationship with your doctor. Being able to discuss what's happening in your life, your fears, your concerns, your changing needs, and issues you don't understand, can be very satisfying. During a routine office visit there usually are too many medical issues that fill the scheduled encounter. Having a visit to "just talk" and keep your doctor informed about what's happening in your life refocuses each of you on what is important in your life, gives you a common agenda, and defines your personal needs. You and your doctor can talk together as two human beings, with the same motivation and concerns: are you doing all right, or should any changes be made? It brings back an important aspect of health care that was lost decades ago.

There will probably be an issue of who will pay the doctor for this type of visit. Busy clinics or insurance companies may feel this visit is "not medically necessary" (again an expression of "treating a disease" and not the patient). If the cost of the visit is not covered, you may have to decide how much such a visit is worth to you. You may also have to become more active in making your needs and demands known, and pressuring your insurance company or the clinic to change their policies. Better understanding between you and the doctor actually saves money in the end, by reducing testing and treatments that may not be necessary.

New directions in therapy

Over the recent decades, medical care and therapy has changed dramatically. In the past, when the more advanced elderly where young, medical care was "paternalistic"; that is to say that the doctor was usually masculine, and treated the patient much like a father figure might treat a child; he did what he thought best without getting involved in discussion with the patient. There was a prevalent attitude among physicians that patients were unable to understand the nature of their diseases and unable to deal rationally with medical decisions. Indeed, patients were never told of some diagnoses, such as cancer. There was an unspoken assumption that the treating physician would always do "what was best." Consequently, the patients placed their lives and their care completely and blindly in the hands of their doctors. After all, how could a untrained patient or individual know enough to question the doctor?

This "paternalistic" philosophy changed in the 1950s and 1960s into a policy of health care that believed patients should be involved in their own health care. The attitude regarding the best health care is felt to arise from physicians and patients working together. Patients were empowered with patient rights. Particularly, they were allowed to choose what type of care they wanted or did not want. This meant they needed to be educated, and not treated as uninformed children.

Today, since women make up the majority of American graduating medical students, perhaps we should talk about "maternalistic" health care. With the majority of doctors now being women, the delivery of health care is changing. Women are demanding more family time to be home with their children. The health-care model we grew up with, and accepted, was one developed by men for male doctors. We are undergoing a change in this paradigm.

New classes of health professionals have recently appeared in doctor's offices and in hospitals: nurse practitioners (NPs) and physician assistants (PAs). Their role in medical care is increasing throughout the country. Nurse practitioners are trained registered nurses, who have completed advanced specialty training and certification in any of a number of chosen medical/surgical disciplines. They are tested and credentialed by State Nursing Boards, and are licensed to examine patients, prescribe medications, perform simple surgical procedures, and authorize tests and treatments in an independent manner. They work mostly in clinics and facilities where there are also medical doctors, who would be available for more complicated problems that might arise. Nurse practitioners have "provider numbers" that allow them to bill Medicare and other insurance companies independently (without requiring a physician co-signature). Physician assistants usually do not have any advanced or graduate degree, but have taken at least two years of prescribed courses in patient care and basic medical knowledge, and most have bachelor's degrees. They too, are tested and credentialed by state authorities. Unlike an NP, the PA must work under the supervision of a licensed physician, who can allow them to perform simple procedures. They are usually salaried, and paid by their physician employer.

A relatively new concept in health care is concierge or boutique medicine. In this system, a doctor charges an annual fee to each potential patient, allowing them to be one of a limited number of people that he or she will care for. The patient has no other out-of-pocket expense to pay this particular doctor, who will also collect any insurance payments for the medical care provided. By limiting the size of the practice, the doctor promises to be more available and give the patient his or her full allegiance and attention. Contracts are signed and renewed annually.

Another growing trend in medical care concerns physicians "dropping out" of Medicare and all other medical insurance programs – not accepting, nor participating in any health insurance plan. Thus there are no restrictions, nor any regulations imposed by the insurance companies; no forms, no paperwork. Payment for services is purely a private matter between the patient and the provider. No insurance reimbursement will be paid.

With the rising financial burden of health care, and the improved technology and availability of computers, various models of future health care have been proposed. They envision more teleconferencing between patient and doctor. Some have proposed more group therapy based on diagnosis and disease. In these proposals, health care costs could be significantly reduced, with, hopefully, minimal risk to the patient. As discussed above, this might work with the healthier younger patient who has more physical reserve and capacity to heal, but may be more hazardous in the elderly. Again, it is focusing on the disease, and not the patient. Older patients are more heterogeneous as a group, have more complex health issues, and need more individual, hands-on care.

In regard to medical therapy, we grew up in the age of pharmaceuticals and surgery. We used medications that tried to alter processes that were going on in our bodies: like reducing inflammation and activity of inflammatory cells, or coaxing cells to make or not make as much of a hormone, therefore influencing blood pressure or blood sugar. We tried to remove "abnormal" cells with surgery—cutting them out, or burning them out with radiation.

We are now slowly entering the age of "biologics." These expensive medicines are a product of research that has learned the "natural signals" that control cell function. We try to turn on, or turn off, cell activities by providing the proper message. It is like trying to "reprogram" cell behavior: telling cells what they should do, where they should go, and how they should behave. Much like an orchestra conductor controlling the musicians in the various musical sections of an orchestra (telling them when and how to perform a particular musical score), the doctor may be able, one day, to direct the fine-tuning of the body's cellular behavior. A variation of this approach is the growing use of stem cells. Here we introduce stem cells that we hope will repopulate, or replace damaged cells, reeducate cells that have "forgotten" their purpose, or re-supply some missing substance.

This is a new and exciting medical world that we are entering. Biologic and medical knowledge is advancing at an incredible rate. Research is opening to reality new opportunities for treatment that were hardly imaginable only a very short time ago. Nanotechnology is providing health care with smaller and smaller devices that are ever so much more sophisticated and capable of testing or repairing functions that were beyond medical capabilities only a short time ago. If the older person was confused about the older medical world, or is just beginning to understand how it worked and what to expect, the new changes will once again cause anxiety, confusion, and fear. The new knowledge will certainly alter how medicine is practiced. More than ever, people have a need to have some inkling of what things are being done to them and for them, for what purpose they are being done, why the treatments are so expensive, and what they can expect in the future.

There also are new directions in health-care delivery and government policy. Analysis of our health-care policy is beyond the scope of this book, but the aging patient, particularly, is affected by Medicare and government health-care policy. Looking beyond the rhetoric of politicians and the infamous special interest groups, aging Americans need to understand how policy changes can have significant impact on the quality and availability of their health care. They need to speak out and make their voices heard. For most individuals (who are basically healthy), 90 percent of their health-care needs will improve regardless of what type of health care they receive. This is why humans have survived for tens of thousands of years without modern medicine. Modern medicine and good medical care can make a difference in expediting recovery, improving functional recovery, and reducing the risk of complications in these individuals. But, for the most part, people will recover from their acute viral infection, superficial wounds, minor trauma, upset stomach, etc., on their own. The doctor and pharmacist may claim, or be given, the credit for the recovery (and may be entitled to some of it), but the bulk of healing is due to the body's own inherent healing mechanisms. These mechanisms, however, also age, and then, with advanced age, good and appropriate medical care becomes more essential.

Drowning in Information Overload

In today's world, medical information is very accessible; indeed, we are bombarded with it whether we want it or not. Pharmaceutical companies now regularly advertise directly to the consumer, even though consumers need prescriptions to purchase the products. They provide carefully selected information to promote their product, and end with the suggestion that the listener or reader should "ask your doctor!" Sometimes, too much information is dangerous.

Many elderly, or their family members, research each of their complaints extensively on the Internet and health magazines, even asking questions from anyone they suspect may know something about their condition. Books describe good medical care and bad medical care, good medications and bad medications. Pharmacies include literature describing all adverse reactions that can possibly happen while taking a particular medicine. Being informed and being proactive in one's own care is important (as I have been trying to emphasize in this book). However, the patient should work with their physician in a cooperative manner, not independently. They don't have to demonstrate or impress their doctor with how much they know (this will be evident as they discuss their illness with their doctor), and they are not being graded for knowing more or less.

In the hospital, informed consent for procedures is accompanied by detailing all the possible adverse reactions that can happen if the procedure were to be done. All this is being thrown at an older person, who is often anxious and overwhelmed with what is happening to them. Although well intentioned, and legally necessary (to reduce liability), it can be unfair to the older patient. This "information overload" can easily increase anxiety, insecurity, and indecision.

Much of the time the geriatrician spends with a patient is spent correcting misinformation they acquired from outside sources, and assuaging fears. When treating physicians feel patients are making a grave mistake in refusing a test, procedure, or surgery based on something they read, or heard from another person they had talked to, the doctors may try desperately to convince the patients of the value of the procedure and urge or badger the patients into following their prescribed medical recommendations. Although everyone has a right to make their own mistakes, this information overload can backfire and result in patients making decisions based on misinformation. If the patients do not trust the judgment of their doctor, they should get another doctor whose opinion they can trust, but they should hesitate in accepting the opinions of others who may not have the education, credentials, or motives they expect and respect.

Sometimes information overload frightens people unnecessarily. Patients taking "statin" medicines to reduce their cholesterol have been warned about drinking any grapefruit juice or eating a half grapefruit, even though they may have been enjoying grapefruit and taking their statin up to the time of the warning. Patients may be afraid to consume any green vegetable when they are taking the anticlotting medication Coumadin. Others stop eating eggs, or meat, because of fear of becoming more ill. Still others are afraid of consuming any alcohol. Each time a news release tells the public of a newly discovered relationship between a food and a cancer, a number of people panic and change their eating habits. Are these reactions appropriate, or excessive?

Remember, the warnings are only intended as guides for the general public. Even with the same diagnosis, there usually are vast differences between people. If you have a pattern of eating and enjoying certain foods regularly, and you are doing well, you are probably safe in continuing what you are doing. The guiding concern should not be fear that some food or medicine CAN give you difficulties; it should be what is the likelihood that it IS, or WILL be giving you problems. Listen to your body. Obviously, if, IN YOU, something is proven to be causing problems, it might be wise to avoid that "something."

Stated again, people are different, and medical conditions differ between people. Some may have medical conditions that are very fragile, and need meticulous supervision, diet control, and medication management; others may have conditions that are more stable, and can tolerate less intense supervision. It's important to know how well you are doing, and discuss how stable your medical condition is with your doctor. Yes, there may be a greater risk in aggravating your medical condition with certain foods and activities, but as stated earlier in this book, everything is a balance between value and risk. If the balance is working, and not causing you any significant problem, there is no absolute requirement to stop what you enjoy unless something comes along that changes the balance.

SECTION IV — SUMMARY AND CONCLUSIONS

For age is opportunity no less than youth itself, though in another dress, and as the evening twilight fades away, the sky is filled with stars, invisible by day.

HENRY WADSWORTH LONGFELLOW

Fearing aging is counterproductive. It detracts from the focus on living. And what, in fact, is it that we fear? Every age has its difficulties as well as its rewards. To a toddler, the frustration may be to walk and reach a low shelf. A student may feel academic and social pressures as enormous at her particular stage of life. A person just starting out in the work force and in a committed relationship may feel overwhelmed with the stresses of "making it." Later in life we may have the responsibilities of caring for aging relatives as well as for our children. Indeed, every age has its challenges, as well as opportunities for pleasure and reward. At any age, many try to escape from the reality and stress that burden them by one destructive means or another. But, as I had stated above, I believe the goal of life should not be to escape from living, but rather to live and make the most of it.

At different times in our lives, we take stock of who we are, where we are going, and what is important in our lives. As we get older, and while we still can, we need to continue doing this practice. We need to prioritize our values and develop a more realistic perspective of aging, who we really are, and what we really want out of life. For however much time we have left to live, we need to fill our lives with activities that bring us satisfaction. Aging should not be feared, but planned for. It is the one time in our lives we have the time to indulge our whims and pleasures, without the time restrictions imposed by schooling and work. Retirement can be liberating. Aging and retirement can be fun. We don't have to worry very much about saving for the future, nor care too much about the impression we are making on strangers. As long as we remain relatively healthy, older age can be the best time of our lives.

But it is a fragile health we enjoy as we age. Things can change suddenly, and our lives can be altered forever. We cannot fight nor retard aging, and need to make accommodations to the inevitable changes as they occur. Living requires compromises. If we are unable to do all the things we enjoyed when we were younger, there are still lots of things to do that we still can enjoy. As we age, we must make compromises to arrive at the best balance for living the best life we can, to be active and productive for as long as possible. I sometimes remind older patients that they have an important choice to make: they can pull up an easy chair to a mirror and spend the remainder of their life watching their body age; or they can get up out of the chair and live and enjoy the remainder of their life.

Example: When I give an elderly person a blank sheet of paper, and ask him or her to write down the ten best times of his or her life, I find no one lists having had a colonoscopy or a mammogram. They always list events, which were social, and involved their loved ones. Since this list indicates what the highlights of their life were, I advise them to seek more such events during the time they still live. The questions posed to the doctor should not be, "Can I do...?" but rather, "How best should I do...?" People should not give up the things they enjoy too readily, or without a fight. The benefit must be truly significant to pay the penalty of giving up things that would fit on that list.

There is no magical path to successful aging. The rates at which we age, and our life expectancy, is a function of our genetic makeup, our diet, our lifestyle, our past cumulative environmental exposures, and our capacity for recreation, exercise, leisure, and rest. We do better when we have less stress, good social relations with people who care about us, and have access to good medical care. Most of these functions are beyond our control. Financial comfort helps a great deal. We all must do the best we can with the life we have, accepting the limitations and difficulties that seem imposed by who we are and where we were born.

Good and sophisticated medical care is often given the credit for an individual's good health and the longer life expectancy many now enjoy; although this is arguable, there is no doubt that bad medical care is a clear negative risk factor. Most of the credit for good health, however, should be placed on the individual: their genetic makeup, their lifestyle, and their proactive medical attitude.

Successful aging, however, is more than just being healthy and living longer. Successful aging means enjoying one's life and living the most satisfying life one can, regardless of one's wealth (or health). It requires being satisfied with who we are and our understanding of the aging process as it continues to change our bodies and affects our living and our health. Successful aging requires dealing with the ongoing changes in one's body that accompanies aging, and focusing one's energies on those activities that promote and enhance the values of living. It means neither dwelling in the past nor yielding life to the dictates of infirmities.

With advanced age, there is a loss of energy and endurance. Physical needs generally increase, and the older individual in time will need outside help and assistance. Family, friends, or hired help can fill this need. It is often difficult for the older person to recognize and accept the reality of their frailty and the need for outside help; but this need will happen to everyone, if they live long enough. What is needed is an understanding and appreciation of what really is important in one's life, focusing on those aspects that can be changed, accepting those that cannot, and sometimes making the necessary compromises. The changes that are brought on by aging do not mean that life cannot still be enjoyed. The changes mean that serious advanced preparation and planning for the future is needed.

For many elderly, advanced age has become boring and tedious. Life is occupied with repetitive drudgery and mindless chores: daily routines without end, without excitement, without any expectation of change. Challenges are avoided. They may not even be stimulated by the occasional interruptions in this pattern by brief interactions or visits with friends and family. This scenario generally means the individual has fallen into the trap of passive existence, complacency, and not of active living. They may be depressed or overmedicated with sleeping pills and antidepressants.

As previously stated, living should be more than just existing. To my mind, successful living requires "4 active L's" (described on page 22): Living, Learning, Loving, and Laughing. It requires being challenged, mentally and physically, as much as tolerated. Reading, learning new material, picking up new hobbies, developing new projects to accomplish, setting new goals to achieve, active participation in community programs, and volunteering are just some examples of the many types of programs available for the elderly that can keep them interested in living, involved in life, and feeling challenged and stimulated. Moreover, these activities are mostly under their own personal control, and are not dependent upon other people's schedules and preferences.

When we look around us and observe people whom we feel have aged successfully, what lessons can we learn from them? They are not living in the past, but living in the present. They face adversity, hardship, and illness with determination and a plan. They have interests and socialize with others. They keep their minds and bodies busy.

How do these "successful agers" do this? Is it their biology, genetics, or "strong healthy bodies"? Is it their social and family-support network, or is it their doctor and health team? Is it their attitude and outlook on life, their understanding of "healthy living," and their preparations for living as an older individual? Is it just good fortune and happenstance? Successful aging seems to be: one-third biology and underlying health, one-third attitude and preparations made and based on knowledge, and one-third just plain luck.

INDEX

4 Ls of Living: 22, 248

Advance Directive: 209, 212-214

Ageism: 20-21

Allergies: 31, 66, 73, 96, 97, 152, 168, 177. 178. 234

Alzheimer's Disease: 67, 71-73

Anemia: 50, 77

Anesthesia: 43, 62, 164

Angina Pectoris: 78, 90, 163

Anorexia: 153

Anserine bursitis: 153

Anti-aging hormones: 7

Antibiotics: 42, 95, 128, 137, 138-143, 168-169, 174, 191, 208, 229

Aortic Aneurysm: 90-91

Appetite loss (see anorexia)

Aspiration: 96, 130, 134-135, 153

Assisted Living: 161, 209

Arteriosclerosis: 47, 89

Atrial Fibrillation: 43, 47, 79

Back pain: 15, 104-109, 116

Balance Difficulties: 33-35, 51-53, 71, 106

Banking: 158

Belching: 126

Black/blue marks (see ecchymosis)

Blacking out (see syncope)

Bladder Control: 25, 30-33, 135-137

Bladder Infections: 135-137, 157

Botox: 7, 32

Bronchiectasis: 97

Bursitis: 108, 153

Cancer: 4, 7, 26, 52, 81, 98-104, 109, 121, 131, 138, 140, 144-145, 147, 163, 187, 211, 212, 236, 242

Carpal Tunnel Syndrome: 64, 65

Case Manager: 34,160, 161

Catheters: 31, 32, 40, 42, 43, 57, 137-138, 143, 157

Cataracts: 152, 159

Chest Pain: 78, 83, 97, 129, 132

Choking on food (see aspiration)

Cholesterol: 7, 9, 21, 46, 47, 73, 83, 84, 184, 242

Claudication: 89-90

Cognitive Impairment (MCI): 16, 19, 68, 211

Computers vs. Humans: 10, 195, 232-234, 238

Concierge medicine: 238

Colic: 127, 128

Colitis: 127, 137, 142

Constipation: 123-125

Cough: 96-98, 131-133, 133-134, 138, 141, 143

CPAP: 62

Cystitis (see bladder infection)

Decubitus ulcer (see pressure sore)

Dehydration: 32, 41, 56, 58, 69, 88, 123, 135, 146, 147, 150

Delirium: 41, 43, 71, 136

Dementia: 16, 41, 42, 43, 61, 68-74, 75, 77, 147, 153, 155, 158

Dental Care: 153, 164, 168, 169, 193

Depression: 20, 26, 29, 33, 50, 60, 70, 75-77, 153, 155, 156, 162, 163

DHEA: 6, 7

Diabetes: 27, 44, 47, 50, 52, 89, 152, 153, 163, 179

Diarrhea: 124, 126, 127, 137, 141

Diet: 9, 10, 120, 124, 127,128, 162, 165-167, 172, 178-180, 186, 243, 247

Diverticulitis: 44, 127

Dizziness: 51, 55-58, 79, 83, 224

Doctors: 17, 18, 20, 22, 24, 25, 26, 27, 29, 31, 38, 39, 40, 42,49, 61, 55, 56, 60, 63, 68, 70, 74, 80-83, 88, 92, 96, 104, 107, 116, 121-123,128, 131, 132, 134, 135, 138, 140-146, 161, 167, 171-174, 175, 176, 178, 180-182, 184-186, 189, 190, 192, 195, 197, 199, 201, 202, 204-206, 210, 211, 214-227, 229, 231-243, 247, 249

DNR/DNI: 209, 213

DRG: 198, 228

Driving: 22, 24, 29, 63, 159-160

DVT: 42, 87, 97

Dyspnea (see Shortness of Breath)

Ecchymosis: 144

Edema: 10, 48, 84-88, 157, 186, 187

Electronic Health Record (EHR): 227, 233-235

EMG: 108, 110

Emphysema (COPD): 94

End of Life Care: 209, 212-214

EOB (Explanation of Benefits): 198

Estrogen: 6, 7, 118, 122, 146, 163
Exercise: 9, 11, 27, 31, 33, 50, 57,
    78, 82, 94, 95, 96, 111, 113,
    115, 120, 134, 153, 154, 156,
    164-165, 169, 237

Falls: 51, 52, 61, 110, 111,
    168, 196
Fecal Impaction: 122, 124, 125, 153
Feeding Tube: 49, 135, 210, 213
Fever: 98, 110, 124, 128, 138-
    139, 143-144, 223
Foot Problems: 84, 87, 90, 91, 92,
    112, 114-116, 149, 150
Fractures: 51-54, 58, 59, 61, 105,
    107-109, 114, 116, 118, 121,
    122, 157

Gall Bladder Pain (Cholecystitis):
    41, 43, 128, 129, 223, 224
Gangrene: 91, 145
Gas, Intestinal: 124, 126-128
Gastric Reflux (GERD): 96, 122,
    129-134
Generic Medications: 172, 176-
    178, 194
Glaucoma: 28, 159
Growth Hormone: 6, 7

Hair Loss (alopecia): 7, 146
Hammertoe: 114, 115
Headache: 48, 179

Health Insurance: 10, 187-196,
    220, 229, 231, 232, 235, 238
Healthy Living: 23, 35, 161-162,
    220, 249
Health Proxy: 209, 212, 214
Hearing Loss: 29
Heart Attack: 41, 62, 78, 81-84,
    129, 163, 213
Heartburn (see Gastric Reflux)
Heart Failure: 10, 50, 59, 77-81,
    84, 89, 94, 96, 140
Heart Rhythm: 41, 43, 55, 62, 80,
    81, 92, 95
Hiatus Hernia: 121, 129, 130,
    132, 133
Hip Pain: 104, 108, 110-114,
    153, 159
Home Attendant: 33, 42, 193,
    212
Hospice: 211
Hospitalist: 202, 205-206, 208
Hospitalization: 38-40, 77, 128,
    147, 164, 180, 188, 200-208,
    226, 228
Hypertension: 27, 44, 47, 62, 153
Hypotension (orthostasis): 56

ICD-9 Codes: 195
Immunization: 11, 167-168
Impotence: 163
Incontinence: 31, 124, 137, 148

Infarction (see Heart Attack; Stroke)

Infections: 9-10, 15, 31, 41, 42, 43, 58, 70, 77, 78, 88, 91, 95, 96-98, 99, 110, 111, 115, 121, 130, 135-138, 138-144, 145, 147, 148, 152, 153, 157, 164, 167, 168, 169, 174, 187, 208, 213, 240

Informed Consent: 44, 213, 241

Insurance Coding: 188, 196-200

Insomnia: 59-63

Ischemia (inadequate circulation): 43, 45, 69, 70, 82, 83, 89-91, 143, 149, 150

Itchy Skin: 146, 151

Joint Replacement: 109, 114, 142, 169

Kegel exercises: 31

Kidney Problems: 32, 44, 50, 69, 84, 120, 128, 137, 140, 186

Laboratory Tests: 139, 182-187, 198, 199, 226, 231, 233, 234

Lactose Intolerance: 126-127

Leg Cramps: 92-93

Length of Stay (LOS): 208, 228

Light-headedness: 55, 56

Living Will: 212-214

Longevity: 12, 13, 22

Macular Degeneration: 28, 159

Medical Emergencies: 225-227

Medications and Medication Management: 18, 23, 24, 26, 27, 31, 41, 43, 44, 50, 51, 52, 56, 61, 66, 69, 70, 73, 76, 79, 93, 95, 108, 109, 111, 113, 123, 132, 135, 137, 143, 145, 146, 150, 153, 154, 164, 172-182, 194, 199, 226, 239, 241-243

Mental Status Testing: 40, 72

Nausea: 83, 124, 128, 141, 143, 153, 179, 223, 224

Neuropathy: 52, 115

NPH (Hydrocephalus): 71

Nurse Practitioner: 41, 202, 206, 237

Nutrition: 78, 166

Obesity: 44, 152-154

Office visits: 15, 74, 104, 138, 143, 145, 175, 185, 186, 206, 215, 217-223, 225, 231, 232, 235, 237

Osteopenia: 118

Osteoporosis: 51, 108, 116-121, 164

Pain: 3, 24, 25-27, 41, 44, 45, 52, 59, 67, 78, 83, 89-91, 92, 97, 98, 99, 103, 104-110,

110-113, 114-115, 116, 123, 124, 125, 127, 128, 129, 132, 139, 145, 147, 150, 153, 155, 159, 163, 164, 202, 210, 212, 223, 224
Palliative Care: 202, 210-211
Parkinson's Disease: 52, 66, 67, 71, 147, 180
Phlebitis (see DVT)
Physician Assistant: 237
Peristalsis: 124
Pneumonia: 11, 96, 97, 98, 131, 134, 135, 140, 164, 167
Pressure Sore: 147-150
Prolapse: 122, 123
Prostate Enlargement (BPH): 7, 30-32, 136, 163
Pruritus (see Itchy Skin)
Pseudo-claudication: 90
Pseudo-dementia: 75
Pulmonary Embolus: 97, 213

Reaction Time: 16, 51, 52, 159
Rehabilitation: 48, 155-157, 215
Rheumatoid Arthritis: 68

Sciatica: 104-105, 113
Sexual Function: 163-164
Shingles: 11, 145, 168
Shortness of Breath: 80, 94-95, 97, 98
Shoulder Pain: 110-114, 129, 159

Skin Cancer: 99, 100, 121, 144-145, 147
Sleep: 59-63, 70, 73, 74, 75, 92, 93, 123
Sleep Apnea (OSA): 62
Sleeping Pills: 51, 59, 61, 62, 63, 70, 248
Spinal Stenosis: 90, 104, 106
Stretching: 33, 93, 164
Stroke: 26, 41, 45-49, 51, 55, 63, 80, 81, 134, 147, 154, 155, 209, 213
Subacute Rehabilitation: 156
Surgery: 15, 28, 32, 38, 42-45, 62, 64, 82, 84, 104, 109, 110, 111, 115, 116, 143, 154, 157, 187, 191, 203, 215, 219, 239, 241
Swallowing Difficulties: 47, 48, 133-135, 145, 153, 166
Swelling in feet (see Edema)
Syncope: 56, 57

TENS: 27
Testosterone and Androgens: 6-7, 30, 146, 163
Thrush: 145
TIA (Transient Ischemic Attack): 48
Tremor: 66-67
Trigger Finger: 65

Urinary Incontinence: 9, 30, 31, 137

Urinary Retention: 30, 31, 136, 137
Urosepsis: 136

Vagal Reaction: 57
Vertigo (BPV): 55
Vestibular Neuritis: 58
Vision: 15, 25, 27-28, 47, 61, 152, 154, 155, 159
Vitamin D: 116, 119, 120-122, 165, 184

Vitamins: 7, 28, 70, 131, 165, 166, 172, 178, 179, 182, 184

Weight Loss: 89, 98, 128, 152, 153
Weakness: 6, 33, 47, 49-51, 58, 65, 57, 83, 95, 147, 178, 218
Wounds: 9, 42, 91, 145, 240

GLOSSARY of MEDICAL TERMS

Actinic—caused by sun exposure
Adenoma—a benign overgrowth of cells forming a clump
Alopecia—hair loss
Aneurysm—a bulge due to weakening of the wall of the structure
Anticoagulation—slowing the clotting of blood
Arthralgia—pain in the joints
Arthritis—inflammation of the joints
Atrium—a chamber in the heart to which blood returns from the body
Atrophy—a wasting away of a tissue
Bronchiectasis—scarring of the air tubes (bronchi)
BUN—blood urea nitrogen (a waste product of protein metabolism)
Cardio—pertaining to the heart
Carotid—related to the large artery going to the brain on the side of the neck
Carpal—relating to the wrist
Cellulitis—inflammation within the skin
Cerebral—pertaining to the brain
Cervical spine—the spine in the neck
Claudication—pain in the legs on walking due to poor circulation

Cochlea—the organ of hearing in the inner ear

Colonoscopy—looking into the colon

Costochondral joint—the joint where the rib meets the breastbone

CPAP – continuous positive airway pressure

Creatinine—a product of muscle turnover used to measure kidney function

CT—Computerized Tomography

Cystocsopy—looking into the bladder

Diverticulitis—inflamed pouch in the intestine

Dysrhythymia—an abnormal rhythm of the heart

Ecchymosis—black and blue due to bleeding in the skin

Edema—swelling due to fluid accumulation

Effusion—a collection of freely moving fluid in a closed space

Embolus—a clot of blood having floated in the blood causing a blockage

Emphysema—a breakdown of the fine webbing in the lungs

Endoscopy—looking into the stomach or intestine

ERCP—a procedure to view the bile duct via a tube through the stomach

Fasciitis—inflammation of soft tissues below the skin (the fascia)

Fibrosis—scarring

Gangrene—tissue dying due to loss of blood supply

Gastro—pertaining to the stomach

GERD—Gastro Esophageal Reflux Disorder (a cause of heartburn)

GFR—glomerular filtration rate (how much blood the kidneys filter)

Glaucoma—an eye disease caused by too much pressure in eyeball

HDL-cholesterol—the good high-density cholesterol

Hematoma—a mass of blood

Hernia—tissue pushing out of its normal anatomical location

Hepatic—pertaining to the liver

Hydrocephalus—increased water in the brain

Infarct—the loss of blood supply due to blocking of an artery

Keratosis—a growth of cells in the skin

Lactose—the sugar in milk

LDL-cholesterol—the bad low-density cholesterol

Lentigo—liver spots

Lithotripsy—breaking up a stone

Lumbar spine—the spine in the lower back

Lymphadenopathy—swollen lymph glands

Macula—the part of the retina where light is focused

Melanoma—a cancer of the pigmented skin cells (melanocytes)

MRA—Magnetic Resonance Angiography (seeing the arteries by MRI)

MRI—Magnetic Resonance Imaging

Neuralgia—pain from aching nerves

Neuritis—inflammation of the nerves

Neuroma—a benign overgrowth of nerve cells into a clump

Nodule—a lump or mass seen on X-ray

Orthostasis—related to standing up

Osteo—pertaining to bone

Prolapse—hanging out below where it belongs

Pulmonary—pertaining to the lungs

Radiculopathy—inflammation of the nerve root leaving the spinal cord

Renal—pertaining to the kidney

Spondylolisthesis—a slippage of one vertebra over another

Spondylosis—arthritis of the vertebra

Stenosis—tight

Sternum—the breastbone

Thoracic spine—the spine in the chest

Thrombosis—a clot closing off a blood vessel

Thrush—yeast infection in the skin or mouth

Urethra—the tube carrying urine from the bladder to the outside

Ureter—the tube carrying urine from the kidney to the bladder

Ventricle (brain)—communicating lakes in the brain filled with spinal fluid

Ventricle (heart)—the muscular chambers of the heart that pump blood out

Vestibular—relating to the semicircular canals in the inner ear for balance

About the Author—Martin S. Finkelstein, MD, FACP

Dr. Finkelstein is a board-certified internist and geriatrician actively practicing medicine and geriatrics for the past thirty-five years in New York, NY. He is a clinical associate professor of medicine at NYU-Langone Medical Center, in New York City, where he has been teaching medical students, physicians-in-training, junior faculty, colleagues, and nursing staff since 1970.

Dr. Finkelstein graduated from New York University School of Medicine and received his postgraduate training at NYU and Bellevue Hospitals in New York and Stanford-Palo Alto Medical Center in Palo Alto, California. Dr. Finkelstein was a flight surgeon in the US Air Force. He has extensive experience in conducting medical and basic science research, teaching medicine and geriatrics, and in patient care.

Dr. Finkelstein has been cited repeatedly in Castle Connelly's "America's Top Doctors" and in *New York* magazine's "Best Doctors in New York" in the area of geriatrics.

Dr. Finkelstein comes from a family of doctors in which more than a score of family members are, or were, physicians. Dr. Finkelstein grew up in a home where his father, an internist and family physician, had his office. Dr. Finkelstein thus has a rare personal view of medicine as it has been practiced and how it has changed over the past sixty-five years.

This is the first book Dr. Finkelstein has written. The stimulus for writing this book has been the hunger for information about common medical problems he has observed in elderly patients during his many years of practice. Because of his clear and simple explanations, and his views and attitudes regarding health care, his patients have urged him to write this book.